W9-CXM-269

A DICTIONARY OF DRUGS

The Medicines You Use

UPDATED AND REVISED EDITION

Richard B. Fisher and George A. Christie

SCHOCKEN BOOKS • NEW YORK

First published by SCHOCKEN BOOKS 1976
First edition published by SCHOCKEN BOOKS 1972

Copyright © Richard B. Fisher and George A. Christie 1971, 1975
Library of Congress Catalog Card No. 76-12241

Manufactured in the United States of America

A DICTIONARY OF DRUGS

To the memory of
Anne Fisher Holtzmann

Foreword to the Updated and Revised Edition

In recognition of the growing importance of psychoactive drugs both in therapy and in research into mental disease, we have greatly expanded the entries devoted to these substances. The two major classes of anti-depressant drugs are now represented by entries under 'Imipramine' and 'Phenelzine', and the former includes a discussion of the diagnosis of depression. A general entry on tranquillizers has been added, and it incorporates a brief description of anxiety. We have also added a general entry on the hallucinogens. The First Edition omitted all reference to local anaesthetics, an omission that we have corrected with an entry on 'Cocaine' that deals with synthetic local anaesthetics in the same context. An entry on 'Morphine' has been added which incorporates an expanded description of the opiates.

In addition to the psychoactive drugs, we have thought it advisable to add a new general entry on antiseptics. They are one of the commonest classes of drugs, and one that is generally available over the counter without prescription.

Otherwise, we are satisfied with the general principles on which the *Dictionary* was based. It has been accepted widely enough that a new edition seemed justifiable to the publisher as well as to the authors. We are thereby given the opportunity to correct a number of errors of omission and commission that have been brought to our attention by careful readers. To them, we are much indebted.

R.B.F.
G.A.C.

Introduction

When we told friends what we were doing during the writing of this book, they invariably raised their eyebrows at the title. 'Drugs?' they asked, suspiciously, and we learned quickly to explain: 'Not narcotics. Drugs in general – therapeutically useful chemicals, for the treatment of disease.'

Fifty-six such drugs are described in detail. The oldest of them, ephedrine, has appeared in Chinese herbals for two millennia. The newest, cholestyramine, was synthesized in 1965, and the great majority have entered the pharmacopeia since 1940.

Within these fifty-six entries, some 300 chemically related agents are named. The range of the *Dictionary* is further enlarged by seven general entries on important classes of drugs: antibiotics, diuretics, hormones, monamine oxidase inhibitors, prostaglandins, sulphonamides and vitamins. The two indexes at the beginning of the book give the trade names and the common chemical names, respectively, of the 300-odd compounds discussed.* The third index (at the end of the book) lists the diseases they treat.

There are more than 2,500 drugs listed in the 1,400 pages of the *British Pharmacopeia*. Our selection was guided by the criterion that each entry should reflect one or more of three characteristics:

1. The drug is a distinctive type of chemical compound.
2. It has a different and unusual biochemical mechanism of action.
3. It affords treatment for a disease which is statistically important.

*Drugs normally have three names: a detailed, descriptive chemical name, a common chemical name and a popular trade name. Aspirin, for example, is a popular name, although it was once a trade name. Acetylsalicylic acid is both the common and the descriptive chemical name of this drug. Unless otherwise stated, all drugs in the *Dictionary* are designated by their common chemical names, which have the merit of being the same or similar in all countries.

Individual drug entries are in general organized under five headings:

1. The chemical name, discoverer, trade names and methods of administration.
2. The chemical classification, and where it is relevant, the history of the agent.
3. Its therapeutic uses, often with a description of the disease which the drug is employed to treat.
4. Its undesirable side effects.
5. The chemistry and physiology of the drug.

The *Dictionary* is not a guide to self-dosage, and no information relevant to the amount of the drug required has been included. The reader should also note that, for two reasons, very detailed lists of undesirable side effects have been given. First, the side effects of certain drugs appear to be the major concern of the mass media, almost without regard to the fact that on balance, the drug may be enormously beneficial, even life saving. We have, therefore, felt it necessary – and this is the second reason – to set the record absolutely straight by listing all known side effects, regardless of how frequently any one of them may have been recorded. We have always noted which are rare and which are common. But the fact that a side effect is mentioned does not mean that *you* will experience it, no matter how often it occurs statistically. If you are taking a drug, guard against the all too common tendency to discover symptoms which are not there. Your doctor will prescribe only what he believes will help you; he knows your make-up, your illness and the drug, and he will warn you about possible untoward reactions if he thinks a warning is necessary.

The fifth heading, chemistry and physiology, often contains rather more technical language than do the first four. In order to make these data comprehensible, we have followed two lines. In the first place, we have included five entries which define a few of the more important concepts underlying modern biochemistry. These are 'Biochemistry', 'Electrolyte', 'Enzyme', 'Ion' and 'Metabolism'. In the second place, we have made every effort to use words and chemical symbols in such a way that they can be understood by the serious reader no matter how limited his scientific background.

To find out what the drug is for, it is necessary to read only the first three sections of an entry. (The general entries are organized more loosely, but their pattern is similar.) It is our belief, however, that the fascination inherent in the applied science of pharmacology arises from the fact that it lies between and overlaps the more basic sciences of biology and chemistry. Indeed, the *Dictionary* is written for the person who takes a drug and wants to know not only that his doctor believes it will diminish his discomfort or cure his illness but also, why. What is it the compound does inside the body which may make him well?

In so far as present knowledge permits, that is the question we attempt to answer. It has taken just over fifteen years for biology to change out of all recognition as biologists have focused their attention on the intricate chemical behaviour of living things. When James Watson and Francis Crick discovered the structure of deoxyribonucleic acid (DNA), the molecule containing the genes which control inheritance, in 1953, they demonstrated that a cause-and-effect relationship can be established between atomic and molecular events, on the one hand, and gross physiological occurrences on the other. In this sense, they founded the science of molecular biology, a fundamental tenet of which is that all physiological phenomena occur as a result of chemical events. Growth and ageing, the sense of health and well-being, the shape and size of organs and the experiences of the senses, according to the theory, stem from scientifically predictable combinations and recombinations of atoms and molecules. Similarly, disease is the malfunction of one or more biochemical balances or processes. Medicine must, therefore, be directed towards the restoration of normal body chemistry.

Drugs provide the connexion between chemistry and biology in two senses: first, a drug is a chemical manipulator designed to set right the biochemical malfunctions which cause the symptoms of disease. Second, drugs can also be tools for the study of chemical balances and processes. If the drug molecule alters a normal chemical process, this change may be reflected in some biological event. For example, in sensitive bacteria, penicillin (q.v.) will halt the biological process of cell-wall construction. With the antibiotic, it has been possible to determine precisely the chemical changes that occur in this biosynthetic sequence. Drugs such as L-dopa (q.v.) were developed as research tools even before their clinical value was recognized.

Some of the entries in this book – amphetamine, cannabis, ethyl alcohol, lysergic acid diethylamide, phenobarbitone – are either legally or popularly classed as narcotics. To that extent our suspicious friends were right. Such drugs can be used for treatment or for research, but they can also provide, however fleetingly, some improvement in the subjective quality of life. Other drugs might also be made to serve this purpose. Some people claim that they can get high on aspirin (q.v.). We have included some narcotic drugs both because they seem to us to meet our criterion of selection, and also because they help to demonstrate a characteristic common to all drugs: they are chemicals. So are our bodies. When the exogenous (originating outside the body) chemical comes into contact with the endogenous chemicals, something as destructive as an explosion can occur. Whether they are narcotics or 'miracle' cures, all drugs can be dangerous. Anyone who takes any drug – with the possible exception of aspirin and some vitamins – under any circumstances other than a doctor's prescription does so at what may be grave risk, to himself and to others.

We have consulted the texts, papers and reports of literally dozens of research workers in order to write these entries, but with the exception of a few direct quotations, they are not acknowledged. Errors of omission or commission are of course ours and not theirs. One of us (G.A.C.) is a practising pharmacologist as well as a physician, and specializes in the field of steroid drugs (see 'Hormone'). As authors, however, we are in this instance journalists rather than scientists. We have aimed for accuracy and comprehensibility, and not for completeness. There is, unfortunately, not space to explain how, when and by whom discoveries were made.

One acknowledgement we are compelled to make, however, in gratitude and affection. The idea for *A Dictionary of Drugs* originated with its first editor, Tony Richardson. He gave the book what shape it has; we filled in the outline. Before we had finished our job, he was killed by a disease which no form of intervention can so far arrest permanently. We are deeply in his debt, for friendship, for foresight and for the optimism which we hope this book goes some way to justify.

RICHARD B. FISHER
GEORGE A. CHRISTIE

December 1970

Index of Drugs by Trade Names

Index of Drugs by Common Chemical Names

17

Acetazolamide

(R. O. Roblin, *et al.*, 1950, U.S.) Trade name: Diamox.
Administration: orally, in tablets or syrup.

Classification

Prototype of a class of drugs known as carbonic anhydrase inhibitors because they delay or prevent altogether the catalytic
action of a common intracellular enzyme (q.v.), carbonic
anhydrase ('Chemistry and Physiology', below). Acetazolamide
was developed from and is chemically related to the sulphonamides (q.v.), a large group of effective anti-bacterial drugs
which preceded the antibiotics (q.v.). The only other compound
of clinical importance similar to acetazolamide is dichlorphen-
amide.

Therapeutic uses

Acetazolamide was synthesized originally as a diuretic (q.v.), and
is particularly useful in reducing body fluid accumulation resulting from heart disease coincident upon diseases of the lungs or
of their blood vessels. Heart disease may well lead to poor
circulation which frequently causes oedema, or the accumulation of excess intercellular fluid. The condition, which can have
other causes as well, may be dangerous because the swelling
presses on organs already weakened by disease.

Glaucoma (excess fluid accumulation in the eyeball) is also
treated with acetazolamide. The drug helps to control the amount
of fluid within the eyeball, thereby reducing intraocular pressure.
For reasons which are not clear, this agent can be used as an
anti-convulsant in epileptic seizures. In recent clinical practice,
however, the carbonic anhydrase inhibitors have been superseded by other diuretics, particularly the thiazides (see 'Chlorothiazide'), but they continue to be useful for research into
kidney functions.

Side effects

Serious toxic effects are infrequent. Large doses may cause drowsiness, and other recorded reactions include fever, skin eruptions, bone-marrow depression and kidney damage and stones. Certainly the most serious condition which can arise from the use of acetazolamide is one called metabolic acidosis, an excessive acidity of the body fluids which can in extreme cases be fatal. An analogous condition called diabetic ketosis (see under 'Insulin') occurs in advanced diabetes mellitus. Reports indicate that in diabetes-prone individuals, acetazolamide treatment over a long period in some cases may have caused the disease. The drug has been known to reverse the salutary effects of chemically related oral anti-diabetics such as chlorpropamide (q.v.) and tolbutamide. Care should be taken, therefore, in the administration of acetazolamide to diabetics receiving these oral medicines.

Chemistry and physiology

Carbonic anhydrase is an enzyme within kidney and other types of body cells. It catalyses the rapid combination or separation of carbon dioxide and water:

$$CO_2 + H_2O \leftrightarrows H_2CO_3 \leftrightarrows H^+ + HCO_3^-$$

carbon dioxide   carbonic acid   bicarbonate

These processes can occur without the enzyme, but they proceed at a much slower rate. As the formula reveals, carbonic acid in turn breaks down into or can be formed from hydrogen ions (q.v.) and bicarbonate. The direction of the reaction depends on a number of variables, including the relative amounts of the three factors available, but not on the enzyme. Drugs that inhibit carbonic anhydrase significantly slow these reactions.

Among the electrolytes (q.v.) affected by the action of kidney cells which contain carbonic anhydrase are sodium (Na^+), hydrogen (H^+) (both of which are atoms lacking one electron – in the case of hydrogen of course, the only one – and therefore showing plus charges), and bicarbonate (HCO_3^-). These cells normally exchange H^+, produced via carbonic anhydrase-catalysed reactions, for Na^+ in the filtrate (see discussion of kidney function under 'Diuretic'), where it is combined with HCO_3^-, as sodium bicarbonate ($NaHCO_3$). Since the effect of the drug is to decrease the amount of H^+ available for exchange, it increases the amounts of Na^+ and HCO_3^- in the filtrate. The acidity of any fluid depends upon the number of free hydrogen ions in it; therefore, because it contains less H^+, the urine is more alkaline than normal. It also contains slightly more Na^+ and HCO_3^-, as well as more potassium and ammonium ion, than the blood plasma outside the cell. The resultant osmotic pressure (that is, the tendency of water to move through a semi-permeable membrane from a less 'dense' to a more 'dense' solution in order to balance them) tends to increase the amount of water retained in the filtrate so that the volume of urine is increased. Gradually, excess body fluid enters the blood and is thus removed from the tissues.

The molecular mechanism by which acetazolamide inhibits carbonic anhydrase is unknown, but the drug molecule appears to bind to the enzyme molecule in such a way that carbonic anhydrase cannot act to combine CO_2 with H_2O.

Actinomycin

(Waksman, *et al.*, 1954, U.S.) Also: Dactinomycin.
Trade name: Cosmegen. Administration: injection.

Classification
The fourth antibiotic (q.v.) to be isolated from a culture of micro-organisms called *Actinomyces*, but now renamed *Streptomyces* (see 'Streptomycin'). Actinomycin D is the least poisonous to human beings of the four.

Therapeutic uses
Despite its relative lack of toxicity, however, the agent is far too likely to damage healthy body cells to permit its use as a normal antibiotic against bacterial infections. It has been most successful in the control of cancer of the kidney called Wilm's tumour which is found primarily in children below the age of five. In the United States, the disease is thought to affect about 10,000 children each year. When used after surgery and in combination with radiation therapy, actinomycin D significantly improves the survival rate. Some patients thus treated remain alive more than eight years after diagnosis. Before the drug was introduced, only one out of twenty patients survived surgery and radiation.

The compound has also produced reduction in testicular tumours, against which it is often given in combination with chlorambucil (q.v.) and methotrexate (q.v.). It contributes to the treatment of rhabdomyosarcoma, a rare muscle-tissue cancer, and affords useful if short-term improvement in treatment of Hodgkin's disease and related cancer-like malfunctions of the lymphoid system, carcinoma of the breast and other cancers. Because of its toxicity, however, the agent cannot be used satisfactorily against malignancies which may require long periods of treatment.

Side effects

The undesirable effects of the drug stem from its cytotoxicity (cyto = cell). Loss of appetite, nausea and vomiting may occur soon after injection. Disturbances of the blood-element-forming tissues can occur even after the drug has been stopped, though this effect as well as the others will disappear eventually with cessation of drug treatment. Bowel problems, inflammation of the tongue and lips, mouth ulcers, loss of hair and skin eruptions are fairly frequent.

Chemistry and physiology

Actinomycin D prevents cell growth and division, thus killing the cell. Its usefulness stems from the fact that the cells of some tumours grow and divide more rapidly than do cells of most normal tissues so that the drug kills more tumour cells than normal cells. The drug consists of complex molecules containing two hydrocarbon rings (see 'Biochemistry') linked by a third ring containing nitrogen and oxygen. The two outer rings are in turn linked to identical polypeptide rings. The triple-ring system (exclusive of the polypeptide rings) gives a yellow-red colour to the molecule and is, therefore, called a chromophore.

Actinomycin D prevents cell growth by inhibiting the transfer of genetic information from the deoxyribonucleic acid (DNA), which carries the genes, to a molecule called messenger ribonucleic acid (m-RNA). Normally, m-RNA moves from the cell nucleus where it is synthesized to the cell's cytoplasm (the material outside the nucleus and within the boundary membrane of the cell). There it becomes attached chemically to tiny intracellular organelles called ribosomes; from the genetic data which have been copied into it as certain specific groups of atoms similar to these groups in DNA, m-RNA determines the amino-acid sequence in proteins synthesized by the ribosomes. Thus, when m-RNA is not formed, protein synthesis is inhibited, and the cell cannot maintain its own life functions.

Actinomycin is thought to interfere with an enzyme (q.v.), RNA-polymerase, which catalyses the formation of m-RNA by moving along the DNA molecule and 'reading' the data it contains. The mechanism by which the drug inhibits RNA-polymerase is not positively known, but evidence supports one of two methods: the drug molecule certainly binds together the two DNA strands which form the double helix of the chromosome at points where one base, guanosine, on one strand, is opposite cytosine, another base, on the other strand. It thus stops RNA-polymerase from moving along the helix either by blocking the helical 'channel' along which the enzyme normally travels, or by intercalation (breaking both strands and inserting itself into the DNA molecule), which also has the effect of halting the progress of the enzyme along the DNA helix.

Adrenaline. U.S.: Epinephrine

(Synthesized: Stolz, 1904, Ger.; Dakin, 1905, U.S.) Trade names: Adrenalin, Suprarenin and over twenty proprietary names in the United Kingdom alone. Administration: injection, inhalation, local application in solutions and ointments.

Classification

A natural body hormone (q.v.) first identified in 1899 as the active agent causing certain effects arising from administration of minced adrenal glands to experimental animals. Adrenaline is the earliest of a large class of sympathomimetic drugs (that is, agents which mimic the effects of stimulation of the sympathetic nervous system; 'Chemistry and physiology', below) which include noradrenaline, also a natural body hormone, amphetamine (q.v.), ephedrine (q.v.) and isoproterenol (see 'Propranolol'), as well as phenylephrine, methoxamine, tyramine, naphazoline and many others.

Therapeutic uses

Adrenaline gives rapid relief from acute bronchial spasms, such as those which occur in asthmatic attacks, and from allergic reactions to drugs such as penicillin (q.v.) or to pollen tests. In combination with local anaesthetics, the drug prolongs their effectiveness, but because of its heart action, it cannot be used safely with many general anaesthetics, including halothane (q.v.), and it is dangerous if used with spinal anaesthetics.

Its constrictive action on peripheral blood vessels makes adrenaline one of the most powerful pressor drugs known. It will control surface bleeding, and can be useful for control of bleeding during superficial surgery and in operations on the mouth and throat. It is of no value in controlling severe haemorrhage, however, nor should it be used to treat shock resulting from haemorrhage.

The drug may restore heartbeat in cases of acute cardiac arrest, though it is usually employed only after other forms of therapy, including physical manipulation, have proved unsatisfactory. Its actions on the heart and blood vessels are so complex that it can do more harm than good in acute heart failure.

Side effects

Because of the complexity of actions exerted by the compound, side effects are frequent and often unpredictable. Because it can cause a sharp rise in blood pressure by constriction of peripheral blood vessels, an intravenous injection can lead to cerebral haemorrhage. Its adverse effects on the diseased or weakened heart occur in part because the drug disturbs the pacemaker centres in heart muscle which control the frequency and amplitude of heartbeat (see 'Digitalis'), and in part because a rise in blood pressure can overload the heart. Thus, asthmatics who suffer from heart disease should be given adrenaline only with the greatest caution. The drug can bring on attacks of angina pectoris in patients who suffer from underlying heart disease. Other untoward reactions may include fear, anxiety, dizziness and weakness, headache and respiratory difficulties, all of which will normally disappear quickly with rest and reassurance.

Chemistry and physiology

Natural adrenaline is released from the adrenal glands in case of non-specific stress situations which elicit fear or 'flight-or-fight' response, but the early belief that it alerted brain, heart, lungs and other organs to cope with such situations is no longer considered valid. At the most, this hormone enhances certain metabolic (see 'Metabolism') activities, particularly in the liver and skeletal muscles, and in relation to the breakdown of stores of fat. Ultimately, it induces cellular activation of an enzyme (q.v.), phosphorylase, which promotes catabolism of glycogen to form glucose (see 'Biochemistry'), the major carbohydrate source of energy in muscle.

Its therapeutic uses arise less from these biochemical actions, however, than from its effects on the sympathetic nervous system. Sympathetic and parasympathetic are the names applied to the two major anatomical subdivisions of the autonomic nervous system, which includes all nerve fibres not under conscious control (i.e. that are autonomous). Among major organs innervated sympathetically are the heart, lungs and bronchi, stomach and intestines, blood vessels and the eye, but all of these structures also contain parasympathetic nerve fibres. Although it has certain applications in anatomy and physiology, therefore, this earlier classification of the autonomic nervous system is less useful in medicine and pharmacology than classification of nerves according to the chemicals which they secrete in order to transmit stimuli across synapses, the microscopic spaces between the ending of one nerve fibre and either the beginning of the next one in line or a muscle fibre cell. Other chemical transmitters will be referred to in connexion with drugs which mimic or block them (see 'Atropine', 'Neostigmine' and 'Pralidoxime' as well as 'Hormone'), but the chemical transmitter which effects the passage of impulses from most, though not all, sympathetic nerves to muscle cells is noradrenaline. Noradrenaline is also the substance from which adrenaline is normally synthesized by cells. The chemical structures of these two catecholamines (so-called because of the two hydroxyl groups on the benzene ring) are:

noradrenaline   adrenaline

Each molecule transmits a nerve stimulus because it is released from the initiating fibre, so to speak, and then binds to a specific receptor molecule on the next fibre (nerve or muscle). The receptor molecule has not been described in detail. The exact effect of the binding of the transmitter to the receptor on the configuration of the receptor is, therefore, also unclear, but that there is a change in the receptor molecule can be deduced from the fact that it causes the cell of which it is a part to respond. It seems probable that the chemical change caused by the bond between transmitter and receptor alters the electrical charge on the receptor-cell membrane.

There appear to be two distinct types of sympathetic receptor molecules, called respectively alpha (α)- and beta (β)-receptors. On the whole, α-receptors are excitatory (they cause the muscle to react by contracting, or if it is normally held in a state of contraction as are sphincter muscles, by relaxing), while β-receptors are inhibitory. There are exceptions to this general rule, however; one of the most important is found in heart muscle which has β-receptors that are excitatory.

Adrenaline binds most readily to α-receptors so that, in small doses, its effects are characteristic of the action of the nervous impulses received by these molecules. But it can also bind to β-receptors, either because the dose is large enough so that the α-receptors are all occupied and some drug molecules are left over for the β-receptors, or because it is applied directly to the latter, as tends to be the case when it is injected directly into the heart or is applied as a nasal spray to relax constricted bronchial muscles.

The fact that both types of receptor may exist in the same organ, and that they may cause either contraction or relaxation, as well as nervous reflex actions set up by any normal muscular response, contributes to the complex and often confused effect of treatment with adrenaline, and other sympathomimetic drugs.

Allopurinol

(Synthesized: Elion, Rundles, *et al.*, 1936, U.S.) Trade names: Zyloric, Zyloprim. Administration: oral.

Classification
Developed in the course of a search for a compound which could slow the metabolic (see 'Metabolism') degradation of a powerful anti-cancer drug, 6-mercaptopurine, allopurinol is closely related chemically to that agent, and to the immuno-suppressive drug, azathioprine (q.v.).

Allopurinol is sometimes classed as a uricosuric because it reduces blood levels of uric acid, and, ultimately, the amount of uric acid in the urine as well. The term is incorrectly applied to this agent, however; it means specifically an increase in uric acid levels in the urine, although the effect of this, it is true, must be a reduction in the blood levels. True uricosurics are, therefore, also useful in the treatment of gout ('Therapeutic uses', below). The most important of these, probenecid (trade names: Benemid, Colbenemid) and sulfinpyrazone (trade name: Anturan) are particularly helpful against chronic attacks.

Therapeutic uses
Allopurinol prevents the appearance of excessive uric acid in the blood of patients who are being treated with anti-tumour drugs such as 6-mercaptopurine. By far its most important clinical application, however, is in the treatment of gout. It rapidly reduces the pain and swelling coincident upon acute attacks of the disease and controls these symptoms in chronic gout.

Side effects
Sulfinpyrazone can have severe gastrointestinal side effects, and can cause allergic disturbances. Both occur less frequently following the use of probenecid. Allopurinol, on the other hand, appears to be almost free of side effects. Rashes, diarrhoea and colic have been reported, and acute gouty attacks can actually occur after initial treatment with the drug.

The causes of gout are unknown. It occurs principally in men, and may be a disease of genetic origin. Abnormally high levels of uric acid, a cellular waste product, are found in the blood of gout sufferers, and it is clear that the characteristic swellings (tophi) are due to deposits of uric acid salts in the affected tissue. (A salt is formed when an acid is neutralized by a base; for example: uric acid + sodium hydroxide → sodium urate + water.) Probably a single crystal of sodium urate is accidentally deposited at the affected joint, and acts as a seed for further crystal formation. The foreign substance produces inflammation, and natural defence mechanisms enhance the inflammatory process. In any event, reduction of uric acid in the blood does reduce urate deposits, the inflammation and the swelling.

In man, uric acid is the final cellular breakdown product of a class of molecules called purines. Of the four bases from which both of the genetically relevant molecules, deoxyribonucleic acid (DNA) and ribonucleic acid (RNA), are built up, two are purines. The last step before the creation of uric acid is also a purine, hypoxanthine. (Uric acid is itself a purine.) Its transformation to uric acid requires the catalytic intervention of an enzyme (q.v.), xanthine oxidase.

The allopurinol molecule is almost identical to the hypoxanthine molecule:

hypoxanthine   allopurinol
(The dotted boxes enclose the differing atomic arrangements)

Because of the similarity, the drug molecule can bind to the enzyme so that it is no longer available to catalyse the breakdown of hypoxanthine to uric acid.

The mechanisms of action of true uricosurics ('Classification', above) are quite different from that of allopurinol. Uric acid is filtered from the blood by the glomeruli of the kidney (see discussion of kidney function under 'Diuretic'), but normally most of it is reabsorbed through the renal tubules. The true uricosurics prevent a large part of that reabsorption.

Amphetamine

(Ebeleanu, 1887, Ger.) Trade name: Benzedrine ('bennies'; also called 'purple hearts'). Administration: oral, injection, spray inhalation.

Classification

Amphetamine is chemically related to adrenaline (q.v.), and is also a sympathomimetic drug; that is, one which mimics the effects of stimulation of the sympathetic nervous system ('Chemistry and physiology', below). Its therapeutic usefulness, however, stems from the fact that it has a powerful stimulant action on the central nervous system (CNS), principally in the brain, while its undesirable side effects arise in part because of sympathomimetic behaviour on the peripheral nerves.

Therapeutic uses

The first clinical use of amphetamine (1935) was to treat narcolepsy, an uncontrollable desire for sleep or involuntary falling asleep. Although it is still employed for this purpose, casual self-treatment with the drug must always be paid for in the coin of fatigue. In narcotic and certain psychotic disorders, the agent serves as an anti-depressant. Parkinsonism and petit mal epilepsy (the less serious form of the disease) may be controlled with amphetamine, and it is part of the antidote for intoxication from an excess of depressive drugs such as a barbiturate (see 'Phenobarbitone'). The agent was among the first to be used for the control of obesity by reduction of appetite, but its side effects, particularly the fact that it is addictive, led to a successful search for other drugs to serve this purpose.

Side effects

In addicts, amphetamine produces depression rather than alertness. Amphetamine is addictive because it may create a psychic craving for the drug. Some authorities believe that addiction involves withdrawal symptoms when administration of the compound is stopped, but if so, they are in most cases mild. Tolerance for the agent develops if it is used continuously, and doses must be increased to achieve the same effects. It is thought that addiction, withdrawal symptoms and tolerance may be interrelated phenomena in that they arise from one or more sequential biochemical events, but the reasons for them are unknown. (For one hypothesis to explain tolerance, see 'Chemistry and physiology', below.)

Large doses of amphetamines can produce convulsions, coma, cerebral haemorrhage and death. In sensitive individuals, doses as low as two milligrams have been fatal. Larger doses usually have less effect after continuous use, presumably because of tolerance for the drug, but amphetamine psychosis can result from chronic employment. Indeed, it has been known to occur after a single dose. Such psychoses are reversible when the drug is stopped. Amphetamine poisoning requires treatment with a barbiturate; if the blood pressure is abnormally high, an α-receptor-blocking drug such as phentolamine (see 'Guanethidine') should also be used.

Other side effects can include dizziness, insomnia, irritability, confusion, hallucinations and increased libido, followed by fatigue and depression. Heart pain and circulatory collapse are among possible cardiovascular effects. Gastrointestinal effects may include nausea, vomiting and diarrhoea. Loss of appetite is due to CNS disturbance.

Chemistry and physiology

Because it lacks the hydroxyl groups on the benzene ring, amphetamine is not a catecholamine. Nevertheless, its molecular structure is sufficiently similar to that of adrenaline and noradrenaline for it to become attached to receptors for the normal neuronal transmitter substance, noradrenaline, in the sympathetic nervous system. (For a detailed discussion of these receptors, see 'Adrenaline'.) Noradrenaline is also a transmitter of nervous impulses across the synapses between nerves in some parts of the CNS. However, amphetamine is thought to exert its CNS effects by combining with receptor molecules for another transmitter substance, 5-hydroxytryptamine (5-HT; also called serotonin). In the brain, 5-HT is an excitant (see 'Phenelzine'); when it comes into contact with the next neuron along the line, so to speak, it causes that neuron to fire. Thus amphetamine may act like 5-HT in the brain; certainly it is a stimulant to brain cells that mediate wakefulness, for example, and it has CNS effects collectively characterized in contemporary slang by the word 'high'. Again, the drug molecule is chemically similar to that of the natural transmitter.

The phenomenon of tolerance may occur because muscle and nerve cells which are persistently stimulated by prolonged presence of the sympathetic amines (noradrenaline, 5-HT, adrenaline, amphetamine) become chemically adjusted to them. The electrical properties of the polarized membranes of these cells would become altered in such a way that more of the natural or the 'artificial' transmitter – the drug – is required to cause the cell to respond.

Prolonged use of amphetamines induces increased activity by two intracellular enzymes, monoamine oxidase (see 'Phenelzine') and tyrosine hydroxylase, both of which play a role in the biosynthesis of noradrenaline (see 'Adrenaline'). Noradrenaline in the brain may be a depressant so that its presence in abnormally high amounts could explain the sleepiness and depression exhibited by amphetamine addicts.

Antibiotic

Literally, a substance which is against life, but in common usage, a substance derived from one living organism to halt the growth of or to kill another. In practice, the category is limited to natural products of moulds or fermentations caused by organisms, or the synthetic derivatives of such products. That natural substances have therapeutic properties has been known almost since the birth of man; many of these are in fact 'antibiotics', but the modern use of the word began with the clinical introduction of penicillin (q.v.) during World War II.

There are now well over a hundred identified antibiotics, but most of them are too toxic for clinical use. Nevertheless, like the earlier sulphonamides (q.v.), antibiotics represent true 'magic bullets' in the sense that phrase was first used by Paul Ehrlich (1854-1915), the Austrian discoverer of the anti-syphilis drug, arsphenamine. They attack bacteria, bacteria-like infective agents (rickettsiae and mycobacteria), fungi and even some viruses, while on the whole they leave mammalian tissue alone. Yet they are by no means absolutely selective, and each antibiotic acts against a distinctive spectrum of 'germs'.

Penicillin, for example, is a 'narrow-spectrum' antibiotic because it attacks a smaller range of bacteria than other agents. Among these bacteria are the causative agents of 'strep throat', bacterial pneumonia, diphtheria, gonorrhoea, anthrax, certain types of meningitis, arthritis and osteomyelitis. Streptomycin (q.v.) and the tetracyclines (q.v.) are 'broad-spectrum' antibiotics because they affect both gram-positive and gram-negative bacteria, as well as some other disease-causing micro-organisms. (Bacteria display a distinctive staining characteristic, identified by a Danish scientist named Gram, which in turn results from the molecular structure of the tough bacterial cell wall.) Still others such as nystatin and griseofulvin are useful only against fungal infections. Actinomycin D (q.v.) is an anti-tumour agent. Two new antibiotics, daunomycin and rifampicin, appear to be the first of this class of drugs to inhibit certain viral infections, including the agent of smallpox. Rifampicin has also proved to be effective against trachoma, an eye disease which causes blindness.

The table* overleaf lists some organisms, certain diseases which they cause and the antibiotics of first and second choice for their treatment.

The selection is incomplete; it has been made to suggest the variety both of available antibiotic agents and of the diseases which these drugs can, in many instances, cure. Penicillin or the synthetic penicillins are far more frequently drugs of first choice than this table implies and in the case of such extremely serious infections as tetanus, no other antibiotic helps at all. Therefore it is of the utmost importance that penicillin not be used indiscriminately because of the danger that resistance or allergy-type reactions to it will develop.

Most antibiotics are bacteriostatic in clinical doses, though they may also be bactericidal in larger amounts and against certain organisms. The former action halts the development of microbial populations whereas the latter kills the infective agents outright. In order to cure the disease, bacteriostatic action by the drug requires that the normal immune-defence mechanisms of the body (see discussion under 'Azathioprine') attack and immobilize remaining bacteria. At least one antibiotic, chloramphenicol, principally a bacteriostat, can display as one of its untoward side effects the suppression of antibody formation.

Chloramphenicol, the tetracyclines (q.v.), kanamycin, lyncomycin, the streptomycins (q.v.), possibly erythromycin and several others act against bacteria by interfering with their biosynthesis of proteins. The exact molecular mechanism by which this interference occurs probably differs from drug to drug, but the end result is suppression of growth, cessation of cell multiplication and eventually death. Unfortunately, all of these agents can also inhibit protein formation in rapidly dividing mammalian cell populations as well as in bacteria. Thus, chloramphenicol suppresses antibody production, and can fatally disrupt bone-marrow production of blood elements because the relevant tissues are in each case characterized by frequent cell division.

*Adapted from Louis S. Goodman and A. Gilman, editors, *The Pharmacological Basis of Therapeutics*, New York and London, 1965, pp. 1176-9.

Organism	Some resultant diseases	Antibiotics	
		1st choice	2nd choice
Staphylococcus aureus	Pneumonia, meningitis, osteomyelitis	Penicillin-G	Cephalothin, Synth. penicillin
(If penicillin-resistant)		Cephalothin Lyncomycin Synth. penicillins	Erythromycin
Streptococcus pyogenes	Pharyngitis, scarlet fever, erysipelas, pneumonia	Penicillin-V	Erythromycin Synth. penicillin
Enterococcus	Heart and urinary tract infections, meningitis	Penicillin-G plus streptomycin	Cephalothin or erythromycin plus streptomycin Synth. penicillin
Pneumococcus	Pneumonia, meningitis, arthritis	Erythromycin Penicillin-G	Synth. penicillin
Aerobacter aerogenes	Urinary tract infections	Chloramphenicol Sulphonamide* Tetracycline	Cephalothin Synth. penicillin
Proteus (not mirabilis)	Urinary tract infections	Chloramphenicol Kanamycin	Streptomycin Tetracycline
Pseudomonas aeruginosa	Urinary tract infections	Colistin Polymyxin B	Gentamycin
Salmonella	Typhoid and paratyphoid fever	Chloramphenicol	Cephalothin Synth. penicillin
Shigella	Acute gastroenteritis	Tetracycline	Cephalothin Chloramphenicol Synth. penicillin
Pasteurella pestis	Bubonic plague	Streptomycin Sulphonamide*	Chloramphenicol Tetracycline
Clostridia tetani	Tetanus	Penicillin-G	
Candida albicans	Skin and superficial mucous membrane lesions	Nystatin	
Treponema pallidum	Syphilis	Penicillin-G	Tetracycline
Rickettsia	Typhus, Rocky Mountain spotted fever, Q-fever	Tetracycline	Chloramphenicol
Lymphogranuloma venereum agent	Venereal disease	Tetracycline	Chloramphenicol

1st and 2nd choice antibiotics are listed alphabetically.
*(q.v.) Not an antibiotic.
Tetracycline refers to any drug of this group.

The penicillins (q.v.), cephalothin and several other drugs act principally as bacteriostats by interfering with the formation of or by destroying bacterial cell walls (the latter action is of course bactericidal). Again this mechanism is not fully understood, and probably differs from agent to agent (for some details, see 'Penicillin'). Bacterial cell walls are rigid structures surrounding the cell membranes; mammalian cells, among others, are surrounded by membranes and not by walls. Thus, most of this class of antibiotic are highly selective against disease-causing organisms because they tend to leave host tissues unharmed. Their side effects are on the whole less frequent and milder.

Another group, including the polymyxins, colistin, gentamycin and nystatin affect the cell membrane to weaken it so that it breaks, or to alter its characteristics with respect to substances it admits to or excludes from the cell. These drugs are bactericidal. For example, polymyxin B is a polypeptide molecule (see 'Biochemistry') containing chemical groups some of which are lipophilic (roughly, fat-loving) and others, lipophobic. Detergents and soaps break films of grease because they contain similarly acting chemicals. Since cell membranes contain lipid (the major constituent of fat or grease) molecules, as well as proteins, polymyxin B is thought to disorient the normal molecular arrangements of the membrane so that cell content escapes. Naturally the organism dies, but so, unfortunately, do host cells. Side effects, including pain from injection, central nervous reactions such as dizziness, drowsiness and impaired motor responses, and kidney disturbances are, therefore, fairly common. Colistin can produce partial deafness and blood disorders as well. These drugs are in other words so toxic that they are only used when the patient will otherwise almost certainly die of the disease.

A final small group of antibiotics, including actinomycin D (q.v.), daunomycin and rifampicin, act by interfering with bacterial biosynthesis of ribonucleic acid (RNA). These agents are bacteriostatic, and like the drugs which affect protein synthesis and cell membranes, may also seriously disrupt host cells, especially those which grow and divide rapidly.

All antibiotics may stop working after extended use. They no longer exert anti-bacterial action because bacteria (or fungi, rickettsia and mycobacteria) develop resistance to them. Drug resistance is an all too common phenomenon which actually means different things with different agents. In the case of antibiotics, however, the phrase refers to the behaviour of the infective agent, and appears to take one of three forms.

Certain bacteria can be induced by an antibiotic to synthesize a new enzyme (q.v.) not previously found in the organism, which literally destroys the drug molecule. Penicillin (q.v.) induces an enzyme called penicillinase, and cephalothin similarly directs the organism to manufacture cephalospirinase.

However, only a portion of any bacterial population possesses the capacity to produce a drug-destroying enzyme, although it is now believed that in almost every population, a few mutants contain drug-resistant characteristics such as the inducible anti-antibiotic enzyme or some other quality as part of their genetic inheritance. Under the influence of the drug, those bacteria which do not possess the necessary 'defensive' characteristics die, and thus the mutated 'resistant' minority are enabled to grow and prosper.

More recently, a third mechanism of drug resistance has been identified. In order to survive, a bacterium must contain genetic information which permits it to defend itself against antibiotic attack. Even within the same species, only a few individuals appear to possess the requisite genetic qualifications, but there is visual microscopic evidence that these 'outlaws' can, under conditions which are not fully understood, actually transfer bits of their own genetic material to other bacteria of the same, and of *different* species. Indeed, it is now believed that bacterial species which infect only animals other than man can transfer their drug-resistant genes to individuals of a related species which do infect human beings. The genetic material that transfers resistance appears to be a species of DNA (see 'Biochemistry') distinct from the single bacterial chromosome, and has been given the name R-factor.

It appears that widespread use of antibiotics in animals as well as in man has encouraged the appearance of resistant bacterial strains, and that these can cause infections in patients who have themselves never been treated with the drugs. The early 1969 outbreaks of drug-resistant enteric diseases, particularly in infants in United Kingdom hospitals, are thought to have been due to strains of bacteria which mutated because they 'picked up' the necessary genes from other individuals in the microbial population.

Antibiotic resistance is now a frequent and often frightening phenomenon. An actual majority of the very high number of gonorrhoea infections among United States troops in Vietnam have been resistant to Penicillin-G. Drugs which act by similar mechanisms, for example cephalothin, show cross-resistance: that is, organisms resistant to one are frequently resistant to both.

New agents are of course introduced to control and kill these mutated bacteria (see discussion of synthetic penicillins under 'Penicillin', as well as 'Streptomycin' and 'Tetracycline'), and combinations of the older agents are also employed. Such combinations attempt to exploit the different mechanisms of action of various drugs because few infective agents are so flexible that they can alter their biochemical behaviour in more than one or two particulars. Combination therapy introduces new problems, however, such as the added danger of combination side effects. Understandably, the greatest caution must be exercised in the administration of antibiotic (or any other drug) combinations when the individual agents can produce disastrous effects. Even more to the point, antibiotics must be used only when no other drug can significantly reduce suffering or save life, and never without a doctor's explicit approval.

Antiseptic

The word means literally 'against infection'. It embraces those drugs that kill or prevent the growth of bacteria, fungi, viruses and other micro-organisms, and that can be applied topically to the body. Strictly speaking, drugs that kill or prevent the growth of micro-organisms on or in non-living things are called disinfectants, and they are not discussed.

Long before the germ theory of infection and disease was established in the late nineteenth century, antiseptic chemicals were used, principally for the prevention of wound suppuration. Iodine, still perhaps the most effective antiseptic, entered medical practice in France in 1839, and was used during the U.S. Civil War. Chlorine in the form of chlorinated lime was used by the Austrian physician, Semmelweiss, to combat childbed fever during the 1850s. Phenol or carbolic acid provided the foundation for Lister's dramatic antiseptic surgery in

Drug	Chemical class	Mechanism of action	Therapeutic use (modern)	Side effects and disadvantages
Phenol (carbolic acid)	Phenol	Denatures protein. Presumably, drug attacks both structural and enzyme (q.v.) protein in germs, but does less damage to body protein	Cauterization of small wounds, dog- and snake-bite	Severe tissue damage
Hexylresorcinol Trade names: Contraceptive creams: Rendell Durachreme Sucrets	Phenol	As Phenol	Disinfects superficial wounds, mouth and throat; use against worms; spermicide; urinary tract infections	Irritating to tissue; some allergic reactions
Hexachlorophene (U.S.: Hexachlorophane) Soaps: Gramophen, Cidal Catox, Sebbix, Ster-Zac, Zalpon Creams, etc.: Bidex, Disfex, Phisohex, Hexabalm, Pologel, Steriloderm, Zeasorb	Phenol	As Phenol	General antiseptic against most micro-organisms. Reduces body odour	Takes time to act; has been associated with dermatitis, brain damage, particularly in infants. Mildly toxic if ingested
Alcohol (see 'Ethyl alcohol')				
Nitric acid	Acid	Hydrogen ions (q.v.) released making the medium too acid to	Immediate cauterization of severe wounds	Severe tissue damage

36

Boric acid	Acid	support micro-organisms (or other life if strong acid)	Skin and mucus membrane infections; e.g. eczema, burns, bedsores	Weak: inhibits growth but seldom kills germs
Iodine	Halogen	Unknown	Kills most micro-organisms. Disinfects skin, wounds, contaminated water	Poisoning is possible by ingesting large amounts. Rare allergic reactions
Hydrogen peroxide	Oxidizing agent	Alters characteristics of membranes or other cell structures	Cleaning wounds; controls vaginal infections; mouthwash	Germicidal action brief, relatively weak. Frequent use as mouthwash may cause tongue damage, but reversible. Use in closed body cavities dangerous
Mercurochrome (U.S.: Merbromin)	Metal	Unclear, but mercury in drug may inhibit sulphur-containing enzymes (q.v.)	Doubtful	Halts bacterial growth, but weak bactericide
Silver nitrate	Metal	Silver causes denaturation of protein	Cauterization; wart removal; used as eyewash against blindness caused by gonococci in infants	Stains tissue black temporarily
Benzalkonium chloride Trade names: Calaxin, Drapolene, Empiquat BAC, Hyamine, Marinol, P.R.Q., Roccal (U.S.: Zephran)	Surface-active agent	Unclear, but may be due to changes in characteristics of cell membrane permitting loss of enzymes (q.v.) and other chemicals involved in metabolism (q.v.)	Pre-operative disinfection of skin; superficial wounds; fungal infections; superficial mouth and throat infections; eye infections	Antagonized by soaps; forms films over surfaces beneath which bacteria can live; can cause poisoning if ingested in large amounts (1–3 g.)
Nitrofurazone Trade name: Furacin	Furan derivative	Unknown, but may interfere with enzymes (q.v.) necessary for growth	Superficial wounds; skin diseases; eye infections	Some allergy-like reactions; mild poisoning if ingested

1865. It is hard to overstate the importance of antisepsis and of the germ theory in modern medicine. Yet there has been overstatement in the matter of antiseptic drugs.

The ritual cleansing practised by western populations embodies risks as well as grotesque waste of time, money and energy. For example, mercurochrome or some other relatively ineffective antiseptic may be used on a wound in the mistaken belief that it can prevent tetanus, among other infections. Not only are disease-causing organisms thus allowed to enter the body, but more important, the patient may have overlooked the only certain way of preventing tetanus: immunization against the disease. Serious wounds, accidental and surgical, are not well protected against infection by any known antiseptic. These drugs do not penetrate living tissue effectively, they are often destroyed by body fluids, and they can damage the tissue they touch. Antibiotics (q.v.) are today the most satisfactory 'antiseptics'.

There are three good reasons for the use of topical antiseptics, however. First, they can prevent infections by micro-organisms that are resistant to or unresponsive to antibiotics. Second, they can be used for less serious injuries, and thus spare antibiotics and reduce the threat from the emergence of new resistant bacteria. Finally, they can be self-administered. Antiseptics may be preferred to antibiotics, moreover, for the treatment of certain urinary tract infections, but in such cases, the drugs are always those prescribed by a doctor.

The foregoing chart describes some of the more common antiseptic compounds.

Aspirin

(Synthesized: 1899, Dreser, Ger.) Chemical name: acetylsalicylic acid. Administration: oral.

Classification

One of a group of chemicals called salicylates. The basic compound, salicylic acid, was derived (1838) from willow bark (*Salix alba*) which had been used for centuries to reduce fever. Oil of wintergreen (methyl salicylate) and salicylamide are closely related compounds with many of the same properties as aspirin. The latter word comes from *spirsäure*, which means salicylic acid in German.

Therapeutic uses

According to one textbook, 'over 27 million pounds of aspirin are consumed yearly in the United States (sufficient to treat over 17 billion headaches)'.* No doubt its analgesic (i.e. pain-killing) effect is the most familiar attribute of aspirin. Although only low-intensity pain is responsive to the drug, scientifically controlled experiments demonstrate that it does raise the pain threshold in the brain control centre. However, to obtain the limited relief it can give, the drug must be swallowed; aspirin gargles to relieve sore throat, for example, have no rational use.

Aspirin is an antipyretic (an agent which lowers body temperature), but only when the temperature is above normal. Its analgesic and antipyretic effects may reduce cold symptoms, but it is not a cold 'cure'. The drug may be as helpful as the steroid hormones (q.v.) for the control of rheumatic pain stemming from swelling and inflammation, and it is very useful in the relief of the inflammatory symptoms of rheumatic fever, but again, it is not a cure. Aspirin can act as a uricosuric (see 'Allopurinol'), and is therefore used to reduce the pain and swelling of gout, but newer drugs serve this purpose more effectively and more safely.

Side effects (also 'Chemistry and physiology', below)

If only because it is so readily available and commonly used, aspirin can be extremely dangerous, especially to children. The major symptoms of mild salicylate intoxication include headache, dizziness, auditory and visual disturbances, confusion, drowsiness, sweating, thirst, rapid breathing, nausea, vomiting and diarrhoea. If the poisoning continues, greater central nervous effects may be noted, including a kind of 'high' without euphoria, along with skin eruptions. Growing acid-base imbalances in body fluids can lead eventually to depression, coma and death resulting from respiratory failure. Other gastrointestinal effects may include mild to severe haemorrhage.

Although it is unlikely that side effects will occur if printed dosage instructions are observed, some people respond badly even to low doses. Strong allergy-type reactions are possible.

* Goodman and Gilman, *op. cit.*, p. 326.

Children dehydrated because of fever can be very prone to aspirin poisoning. People with certain forms of kidney disease, and patients taking cocaine (q.v.), morphine (q.v.) or other central nervous system (CNS) depressants – including alcohol – should be extremely cautious with aspirin, itself a potential depressant. No certain evidence exists of aspirin tolerance which would require increased doses, at least with respect to the antipyretic and analgesic effects of the drug. It shows no greater pain-killing properties in combination with other compounds such as caffeine, phenacetin, acetaminophen or salicylamide, furthermore, than does aspirin alone.

Chemistry and physiology

The chemical structure of the molecule is extremely simple:

$$COOH \qquad\qquad COOH$$
$$OCOCH_3 \qquad\qquad OH$$

aspirin (acetylsalicylic acid)   salicylic acid

It is thus an ester (see 'Biochemistry,') of acetic acid.

Both the antipyretic and the analgesic effects were for many years thought to be central; that is, the drug somehow affects the temperature control centre (the hypothalamus) and the pain centre (subcortical regions, probably the thalamus) of the brain. More recently (6/71), however, a new hypothesis of action has been advanced. The drug almost certainly acts locally to reduce inflammation by blocking cellular biosynthesis of certain prostaglandins (q.v.) which mediate this defensive reaction against invasive substances.

In addition to the antibody-antigen immune response mechanisms (see discussion under 'Azathioprine'), cells in various tissues including the lungs participate in defensive reactions by synthesizing and releasing a number of agents which cause peripheral blood vessels to open. More blood flows through the tissue and more fluid collects in its intercellular space. The blood and fluid contain antibodies, lympho-cytes, leucocytes (white blood cells) and other primary defensive artillery, so that the heat, swelling and pain which result from engorgement of the tissue reflect a secondary defensive mechanism: the chemicals released by the cells.

These substances include histamine, certain other 'local' hormones (q.v.) called kinins and prostaglandins (q.v.), and at least three unidentified chemicals. It is possible that they appear in sequence, each one triggering the next in what is called a cascade effect. An analogous series of events is seen in the process which produce blood clots (see 'Dicoumarol' and 'Heparin'). Such elegant and intricate cascades, in which the appearance of chemical A causes cells to synthesize chemical B (other factors being equal) causing cells to synthesize chemical C (other factors being equal) and so on, through a dozen or more steps, are another form of biophysical defence. The fibrin found in blood clots and the final chemical in the secondary defence chain are powerful substances capable of stopping the flow of blood or causing generalized inflammatory reaction, respectively. In other words, they are potentially deadly poisons. The cascade thus represents another mechanism by means of which the body protects itself against itself, so to speak.

Though the evidence that aspirin prevents formation of prostaglandin is strong, its molecular mechanism of action remains unclear. The immediate precursor out of which cells synthesize the local hormone (q.v.) is arachidonic acid, and it is probable that the aspirin molecule competes with this substance for the active site in the enzyme (q.v.) that catalyzes formation of prostaglandins.

Whether this action has any relation to the analgesic and antipyretic effects of the drug is also unclear. A prostaglandin injected into the brain of a cat causes fever, a fact which is compatible with the hypothesis that the substance mediates central temperature control. There is also some evidence that headache can be caused by a prostaglandin, but pain can occur for many other reasons.

However it occurs, the antipyretic effect of aspirin is accompanied by sweating, although only if the patient has a fever. As body temperature falls, metabolic (see 'Metabolism') rate also declines. It will rise again if the dosage is maintained because aspirin tends to cause an increase in oxygen consumption. In toxic doses, the drug partially reverses its effects to produce fever, more sweating and dehydration.

Oxygen consumption may increase because aspirin disrupts a vital intracellular biochemical process which occurs in two stages, and is called oxidative phosphorylation. Normally, oxygen atoms contribute to the biosynthesis of ATP, the energy-storage molecule (see 'Biochemistry,'). Acetylsalicylic acid is thought to uncouple the first stage – oxidation (either the removal of hydrogen from or the addition of oxygen to a molecule, or both) which is a source of energy for the building up of ATP molecules – from the second stage phosphorylation, in which phosphates utilizing the energy from oxidation are bound esterically to adenosine nucleoside (see 'Vitamin', Notes on table – Vitamin B_2). The cell is left spinning its wheels unproductively. More oxygen atoms are required because the oxidative process speeds up in an attempt to compensate for the failure to produce ATP.

The uncoupling of oxidative phosphorylation could help to explain other metabolic effects of aspirin. Thus, it inhibits the biosynthesis of hyaluronic acid, a substance most frequently found in connective tissue which slows the spread of fluids, infective agents and inflammatory substances. These can then build up locally with resultant inflammation, swelling and pain. Reduction in the tissue content of hyaluronic acid would contribute to the anti-inflammatory effects described above, and to the anti-rheumatic benefits obtained from the drug.

Rheumatic fever and certain other rheumatic disorders, however, are also thought to be associated with disturbances of the immune-response mechanisms themselves. There is evidence that these primary defences against invasion sometimes produce antibodies which attack the body's own tissues, thus causing disease. Aspirin does suppress antibody production so that it could act directly against the cause of these so-called 'auto-immune' diseases.

An entirely different category of metabolic reactions is associated with the increased oxygen consumption mediated by aspirin. Breathing is stimulated because the drug indirectly excites the respiratory control centre in the medulla of the brain. Uncoupling of oxidative phosphorylation increases the amount of carbon dioxide in the blood, and abnormal quantities of this gas trigger nerves in the neck which are chemically sensitive to it. These chemoreceptors in turn stimulate the medulla. However, large doses of the drug tend to depress the medulla, as well as other brain centres. As a result, breathing slows down, thus contributing to a further rise in blood CO_2. Because the carbon dioxide causes blood and other body fluids to become more acid, a condition known as respiratory acidosis ensues, and may be accompanied by metabolic acidosis. The combination can be fatal.

In fact aspirin evokes very complex responses in the delicate balancing mechanisms which normally maintain body fluids within a narrow acid-alkali range. Thus the respiratory and metabolic acidoses are only the other extreme from an initial alkalosis which the drug may also cause. While the alkalosis may itself be seriously detrimental, it has at least one particular effect on the usefulness of aspirin itself. The desirable uricosuric actions of the drug occur because it seems to inhibit tubular reabsorption of uric acid. This action is increased if the urine is more alkaline than normal.

It remains to note that aspirin can damage the mucosal cells which line the stomach. Again the reason is unclear. Buffered aspirin (i.e. aspirin combined with an alkali such as sodium bicarbonate) may diminish the risk of such damage. Because of the danger, however, as well as because of factors related to solubilization of the drug and to the clearing of food through the stomach, aspirin tablets should be swallowed dissolved in amounts of water, and should not be taken on an empty stomach.

Atropine

(Isolated: Mein, 1831, Ger.) Trade names: derivatives and salts of atropine have been given trade names, but the compound itself is known either as atropine or as belladonna. Administration: oral, injection, eye-drops.

Classification

Originally purified from deadly nightshade, *Atropa belladonna*, the belladonna drugs, atropine and scopolamine, are found in a wide range of plants, preparations from which have been used for centuries by physicians, and as poisons. They are natural alkaloids (i.e. basic substances, as opposed to acidic, found in plants, usually bitter tasting; they include caffeine, morphine, nicotine, quinine and strychnine). Similar pharmacological characteristics are found in a large class of more recent synthetic agents including poldine methylsulphate (q.v.), oxyphenonium, dibutoline and oxyphencyclimine.

Therapeutic uses

Atropine and scopolamine were for many years almost the only drugs helpful in the control of parkinsonism. In spite of the existence of a large number of new agents for the treatment of this condition, the belladonna alkaloids continue to be employed. Scopolamine has several other clinical advantages with respect to disorders of the central nervous system (CNS), but it is atropine in huge doses which affords drug shock therapy for schizophrenia. The reason for its usefulness against this psychosis is unknown.

When it is used for preanaesthetic medication, atropine reduces salivation and mucous secretion in the respiratory tract. During anaesthesia, it may restore disturbed heart rate and arterial blood pressure; it will also speed up and regularize heartbeat adversely affected by conditions other than surgery. Atropine-induced reduction in the secretions of the upper and lower respiratory tract explain the use of this compound as a common constituent of cold-'cure' preparations. It may also provide relief from severe hay fever and coryza, but it is of uncertain value in the treatment of bronchial asthma.

Atropine affords symptomatic relief from peptic ulcers, though it is normally used with other drugs. In large doses, this agent can relieve certain forms of gastrointestinal spasm, but the side effects of the drug may be more unpleasant than the condition. Related synthetic drugs such as poldine methylsulphate (q.v.) appear to be better spasmolytics.

Side effects

As with all drugs which achieve their therapeutic effects by altering the state of nervous tissue (and a great many whose mechanism of action is quite different), atropine can be a poison. Fatalities are rare, though children are more sensitive to the drug than adults, and the fatal dose varies widely. In part this is true because a limited tolerance to the agent exists; that is, more and more of the drug must be used to achieve the desired effect. However, atropine is not addictive. In belladonna poisoning, the CNS effects are psychotic excitation followed by depression, circulatory failure, paralysis, coma and respiratory collapse. Other effects include dryness of the mouth, intolerance of light and blurred vision, skin rash, rising body temperature (to 109° or more, in infants), weak and rapid pulse with elevated blood pressure and possibly nausea and vomiting. Other side effects are rare, but they can include acute glaucoma, and impotence in younger men.

Chemistry and physiology

Atropine acts as a parasympathetic blocking agent. The parasympathetic nervous system is one of the anatomical subdivisions of the autonomic nerves, the other being the sympathetic (see 'Adrenaline'). In general, parasympathetic nerves communicate commands opposite to those transmitted by the sympathetic fibres. Thus, whereas sympathetic beta-receptors in the heart are excitatory, the parasympathetic innervation inhibits heart action.

From the standpoint of medicine and pharmacology, the more useful distinction among nerve systems is made on the basis of the chemicals secreted by neurons which transmit stimuli across nerve synapses or between nerve ends and muscle. As in the case of the sympathetic nerves, with their alpha- and beta-receptors, so also parasympathetic nerves appear to have two types of receptor molecules for the transmitter chemical. One such type can be stimulated by nicotine, the other by a drug called muscarine. Neither drug is found naturally in the body, of course, and both are used experimentally for the purpose of determining the class of parasympathetic receptor on nerve or muscle cells in various tissues.

Atropine and all compounds related to it are anti-muscarinic drugs; they inhibit the action of the natural parasympathetic nerve-muscle transmitter at the muscarinic receptors. The transmitter is a chemical called acetylcholine (ACh). Muscarinic receptors are located in the eye, the bronchi and bronchioli, the heart and major arteries, salivary glands, stomach and gut and the bladder, as well as in other tissues and organs. Very high doses of atropine will also inhibit transmission by ACh at non-muscarinic receptors in certain ganglia (plural of ganglion; the sub-station switchboards of the nervous system, varying in size and importance but much smaller than the brain and spinal cord), and possibly at muscles under voluntary nervous control as well.

The belladonna alkaloids are esters (see 'Biochemistry,') of tropic acid and either tropine (in atropine) or scopine (in scopolamine) which are organic bases:

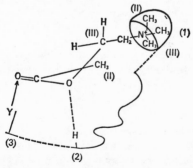

In order to inhibit normal transmission of nervous impulses across synapses, the drug molecule must bind chemically to the receptor molecule, thus excluding the natural transmitter. To know how this happens, it is necessary to know the chemical content and structure of the receptor. Enough information is available about the receptor molecule for ACh so that its approximate portrait may be drawn (see formulae below).

The outline is intended to represent the receptor within which the acetylcholine molecule lies. Note that the space represented is three-dimensional, though only the 'cap' of the receptor (1) is shown in perspective. The dotted lines in the receptor outline indicate areas of uncertainty, whereas the dotted line between H on the receptor and O in the ACh molecule (2) represents a type of chemical link called a hydrogen bond. This bond is thought to be important for muscarinic action, whereas the bond indicated by the arrow at (3) is thought to

be more significant for nicotinic action. More recent evidence (1/70) supports this general description of the bonds between transmitter and receptor molecules for muscarinic and nicotinic action, respectively, with this additional information: the muscarinic bond at (2) also involves the groups marked (II), and the nicotinic bond at (3) also involves the groups marked (III). (A dissimilar hypothesis was advanced eight months later.) The receptor group of atoms in the cap at (1) is believed to consist of several phosphate molecules, a polyphosphate, to which the relevant portion of the ACh molecule is bound by another type of electro-chemical force, related to the negative charge (−) on the cap and the positive charge (+) on the N in the ACh molecule.

Even this much information about the structure of biological molecules other than enzymes (q.v.) and certain formed elements of the blood (such as red blood cells) is unusual. Yet it is still not possible to say exactly how the atropine molecule, the shape of which is of course also known, prevents the muscarinic bond between the receptor and ACh (at 2) from forming. It is known that atropine is a competitive antagonist to ACh; that is, the drug is bound to the receptor more firmly than ACh, so that the atropine-receptor complex dissociates less rapidly than the ACh-receptor complex. However, increased amounts of ACh at the site will overcome the atropine, because relatively more ACh molecules thus become available to the receptors, and nervous stimuli will again be transmitted normally across the synapse.

Azathioprine

(Hitchings and Elion, 1957, U.S.) Trade name: Imuran.
Administration: oral.

Classification
One of a class of tissue-destroying drugs (see 'Chlorambucil', 'Methotrexate') developed in a successful attempt to slow the metabolic (see 'Metabolism') breakdown of a powerful anti-cancer drug, 6-mercaptopurine, to which azathioprine is chemically related. Allopurinol (q.v.) also has a similar molecular structure.

Therapeutic uses
Azathioprine has been employed with some success in the treatment of leukaemia, although it affords no longer periods of relief from symptoms of the disease than does 6-mercaptopurine or other anti-tumour drugs. Its major application has been in the suppression of the normal immune responses. This immuno-suppressive role explains the use of the drug during and after organ transplantation, as well as for treatment of a class of illnesses called auto-immune disease. These include certain anaemias, some kidney disorders and rheumatoid arthritis.

Side effects

Unwanted actions of azathioprine occur because the drug suppresses growth of cells in healthy tissue as well as in tumours ('Chemistry and physiology', below). Thus, by suppressing the growth of cells which are responsible for the maintenance of immunological defences against bacteria and other potential foreign invaders of the body, it opens the way to infection. It can also retard the formation of blood cells by bone marrow, thus possibly aggravating anaemic conditions which exist for other reasons. Clinical symptoms of these side effects include loss of appetite, nausea, vomiting and bloody diarrhoea.

Chemistry and physiology

The normal immune-response mechanisms help to defend the body against foreign substances and organisms such as large molecules (e.g. protein; see 'Biochemistry'), bacterial poisons and bacteria, viruses and dust particles. Food is broken down by digestive action into usable molecules before it passes through the intestinal wall into the blood. In fact, the only known foreign object normally tolerated by the healthy human body is the foetus, and the biochemical reasons for *this* tolerance are not yet clear.

The principal cells involved in this vital defence function are called lymphocytes (i.e., lymph cells). They produce extremely complex protein molecules called immunoglobulins that are carried by the blood. Within their chemical structure, immunoglobulins contain active and highly specialized polypeptide (see 'Biochemistry') segments called antibodies. Antibodies combine chemically with antigens (foreign invaders, or molecules on the surface of foreign invaders) so as to immobilize or destroy them. Though there are only from four to six types of immunoglobulin in man, antibodies come in thousands of varieties, each one specific for one or a very small number of antigens, that is, for a virus, a bacteria or bacterial toxin or a foreign protein from some other source. Furthermore, it is believed that all antibodies are produced as parts of immunoglobulins by lymphocytes possessing the necessary genetic qualifications upon challenge by specific invaders.

Lymphocytes originate in lymphoid tissue, the glands and tubes that regulate the flow of a normally colourless body fluid called lymph. The tubes conduct lymph from tissues where it is formed, ultimately from the blood, to the blood vessels. New lymphocytes are formed constantly, just as new red blood cells develop in bone marrow throughout life.

When a foreign substance enters the body, it may be attacked by antibodies. If the invader has appeared before, for example because of previous vaccination or infection, the necessary antibodies either exist or can be quickly produced by those lymphocytes that were

47

'tooled up' to synthesize them as a result of the earlier appearance of the antigen. But if the invader is new – for example, a new kidney – one or more lymphocytes may begin to grow and divide very rapidly and to produce immunoglobulin containing new antibody directed against antigens in the transplant. Therefore, at least temporary suppression of these cells is required if rejection is to be prevented.

Auto-immune disease, on the other hand, is thought to appear when the immune mechanisms malfunction. Normally, they will attack only substances foreign to the body. There is much experimental evidence, however, that they do occasionally appear to 'forget' what is 'self', and begin to treat a specific tissue as 'not-self', in the classic formulation of the great British immunologist, Sir Macfarlane Burnet. The result is the destruction of cells in the tissue attacked. The reasons for this malfunction are unclear, though it probably stems from a mutation in the genes of one of the millions of rapidly growing and dividing lymph cells. Whatever the cause, however, it is again necessary to suppress lymphoid cell growth in order to control the condition.

Azathioprine performs this function because it interferes with the biosynthesis of purine molecules essential for the cellular formation of the genetically relevant molecules, ribonucleic acid (RNA) and deoxyribonucleic acid (DNA). The azthioprine molecule contains within it a 6-mercaptopurine molecule, so to speak, which is strikingly similar to a natural metabolite of both RNA and DNA, hypoxanthine. The latter is also a catabolite (that is, a breakdown product of the nucleic acids), which is logical because what goes in may be expected to come out:

azathioprine

6-mercaptopurine

hypoxanthine

In one of the early steps in the biosynthesis of RNA, hypoxanthine becomes part of a molecule called hypoxanthine ribonucleotide, or inosinic acid. Within the cell, the azathioprine molecule is reorganized into 6-mercaptopurine, which can replace hypoxanthine to form 6-mercaptopurine ribonucleotide. The sulphur atom in this molecule causes it to behave differently from hypoxanthine (which has an oxygen atom in the same position) so that correctly structured RNA, and

DNA, fail to appear. Both azathioprine and 6-mercaptopurine probably disrupt other biosynthetic processes, but as far as is known, the end product of all such processes is normally RNA and DNA. Without correctly formed nucleic acids, the cell will cease to grow, and will either fail to divide, or will divide so that the daughter cells contain malformed genetic material and die.

Biochemistry

'The chemistry of carbon compounds' (Kekulé, 1860) evolved early in the nineteenth century as the chemistry of living things. The early organic chemists thought that carbon compounds were exclusively found in living things, and that they were, furthermore, the principal constituents of organisms. Although the former is not true, the latter has some validity.

Carbon (C), the sixth element in the Periodic Table of the Elements, combines to make more known compounds than do all other elements together. But hydrogen (H) and oxygen (O), largely in the form of water, are far more frequent in living matter (both in terms of weight and in terms of the total number of atoms of each), and nitrogen (N) plays a vital, central role in compounds containing one or more of the other three principal elements in life. In addition, traces of other inorganic elements are essential to all living systems; in the order of their appearance in the Periodic Table, these include: sodium (Na), magnesium (Mg), phosphorus (P), sulphur (S), chlorine (Cl), potassium (K), manganese (Mn), iron (Fe), copper (Cu), iodine (I).

Organic chemistry is thus a historically interesting phrase, the meaning of which is too restricted to apply to the modern chemistry of life. This science is now called biochemistry.

Like all branches of chemistry, biochemistry deals with elements and with the laws by which they combine; however, it is concerned only with those elements found naturally in living matter, or used pharmacotherapeutically, in drugs. Thus gold (Au) and radium (Ra), for example, while they are not normally found in living organisms, may be introduced into them in an attempt to correct disease states. Almost all drugs also contain carbon, hydrogen and oxygen; nitrogen and other elements found in life are also in some drugs.

Elements are of course the building blocks of matter in that each of them consists of an atom which differs chemically and physically from all other atoms. An atom has a nucleus, the major components of which are (from the standpoint of this *Dictionary*) positively charged particles called protons, and negatively charged particles (the word is not quite accurate when applied to electrons) which revolve around it, so that the whole atom is analogous to, though not the same as, a solar system. The atoms of each element have a specific number of protons in their nucleus and an equal number of electrons moving about this core. Since it is the electrons which are actively involved in the formation of chemical compounds, it is customary to differentiate elements with respect to the number and location of the electrons their atoms contain. The atomic weights of elements also differ, being roughly twice the number of protons, and this mass is almost entirely found in the nucleus (an electron weighs $\frac{1}{1836}$ of a proton). The Periodic Table, however, is arranged in the first instance according to atomic number (actually, the number of protons in the nucleus), as well as by the location and orbits of the electrons.

Hydrogen (atomic number 1) has 1 proton and 1 electron. Carbon (atomic number 6) has 6 of each, nitrogen 7 and oxygen 8. Although each of these atoms is electrically neutral because the number of positively charged protons balances the number of negatively charged electrons, all four elements are nevertheless highly reactive; that is, they are each capable of combining with another atom of the same kind or with each other (and with most other elements) by means of energy links called bonds (see below). Bonds are mediated by electrons, but only by certain of the outer electrons on each atom. (Hydrogen has only one electron which must, therefore, form bonds between one hydrogen atom and another or between hydrogen and atoms of most other elements, but the actual role of this electron in bonding is often far more complicated than this oversimple description suggests.)

All matter builds up because atoms become bonded together into molecules. These bonds may be strong or weak in terms of the energy required to forge or to break them, but living molecules, the subject of biochemistry, are exactly the same as nonliving molecules from the standpoint of the atoms out of which, and the laws in terms of which, they are made. Thus in theory at least any molecule in a living organism could also exist outside it. Any chemical process occurring inside an organism, whether the process involves the bonding together of atoms into molecules, or changes in the molecules thus created, could occur apart from it.

Biochemical processes are distinguished from non-biological chemical events by the fact that the former supply their own energy. (In physical terms, a living organism appears to run counter to the second law of thermodynamics which states that an organized system is always tending to become more and more disorganized. Living cells create order out of disorder, until they die. Then, the second law intervenes at once.) Thus in a test tube, a molecule of water (H_2O; i.e. two atoms of hydrogen and one of oxygen bonded together via certain electron links between them, although it should be noted that in pure water only a portion of the H_2O exists in this form as molecules: some is always naturally dissociated into H and OH, these particles being held in solution by reason of their positive and negative electrical charges, respectively) may be made to separate into its component atoms by the application of heat, among other techniques. The heat energy breaks the bonds (it is actually converted into a form of electrical energy) between the atoms. Body temperature normally remains constant at $37°$ C ($98.6°$ F), yet water molecules are constantly being broken down (and synthesized) within the body. The energy for these reactions will be discussed at the end of this entry.

Ultimately, its source is the food we eat, the largest part of which is itself the product of biochemical processes. In terms of weight, the major constituents of food are fats, carbohydrates and proteins, though not necessarily in that order. To understand the chemical nature and biological significance of these substances, it is convenient to revert to the idea that carbon is the principal organic compound.

Because of the arrangement of its outer electrons, an atom of carbon will normally combine with four other atoms, including of course other atoms of carbon itself. Thus long chains of carbon atoms may be built up as a sort of backbone along which are attached in the proper number other atoms. The simplest of these molecular structures are hydrocarbons; that is, combinations of carbon and hydrogen:

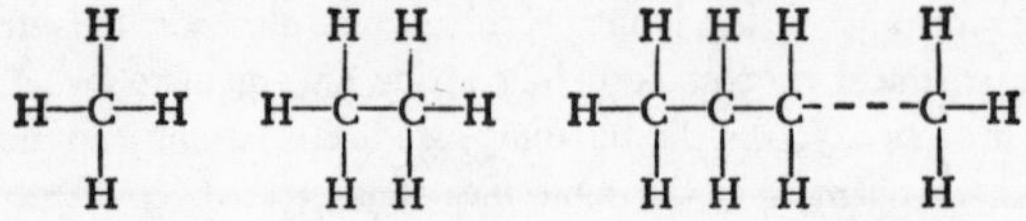

CH_4 = methane C_2H_6 = ethane C_nH_{2n+2} = straight-chain hydrocarbon

Another type of molecular structure also arises from the nature and location of the outer electrons of the carbon atom. This involves a double bond, in that a carbon atom may link itself to certain other atoms twice, and then to only two additional atoms rather than three:

C_2H_4 = ethylene

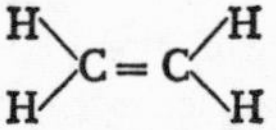

Although this compound is stable in the sense that considerable energy is required to break the double bond between the two carbon atoms, it is called unsaturated because under certain conditions, one of the bonds may be ruptured so that each of the carbon atoms can combine with a fourth atom. Thus in many important biological reactions, the elements of water are added across the double bond – that is, to each of the carbon atoms, H going to one, and OH to the other. This process is called hydrolysis.

Carbon compounds may also be built up in rings rather than in straight-line chains. Particularly common are six-membered rings, one of the most familiar of which is benzene, C_6H_6:

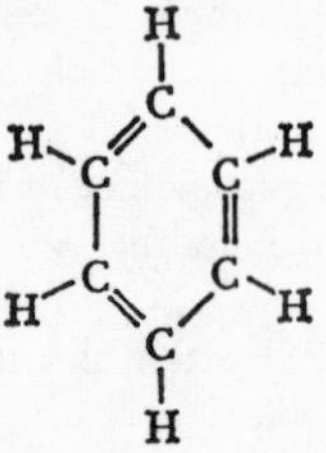

or this may be written,

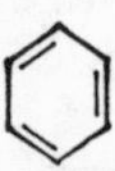

(A)   or   (B)

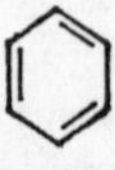

(C)

Note that because carbon combines with four other atoms, the ring contains alternate double bonds (that is, it is unsaturated), but the conventional drawings of the benzene ring shown above are inaccurate; the double bonds may equally well be as portrayed in either (B) or (C). Ring compounds of this type are called 'aromatic' because of an inaccurate nineteenth-century generalization to the effect that all such structures have an odour. Straight-line carbon chains are called 'aliphatic'.

Any of the hydrogen atoms in straight-line or in ring hydrocarbons may be replaced by another atom or group of atoms. In biological molecules, oxygen is one of the most frequent of these substituents.

Among the most important oxygen-containing groups are:

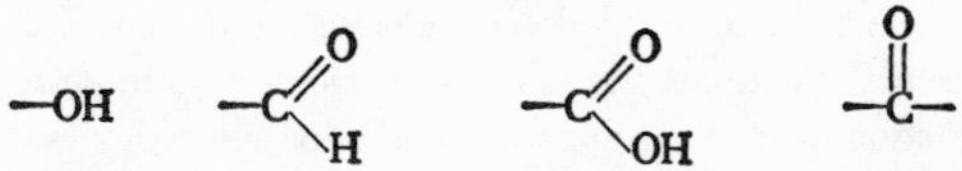

| hydroxyl | aldehyde | carboxyl | oxo or keto |

The other end of the open bonds is attached to other atoms or groups of atoms to form stable compounds. Thus, when a hydroxyl group is added to a hydrocarbon, an alcohol exists:

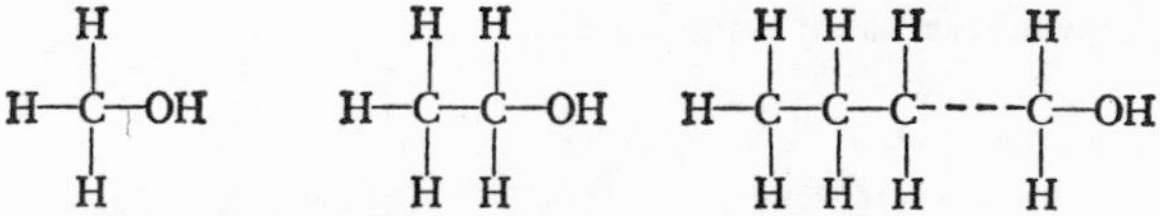

CH_3OH = methanol or methyl alcohol C_2H_5OH = ethanol or ethyl alcohol $C_nH_{2n+1}OH$ = alcohol (general formula)

Carboxyl-containing groups are acids because the group can dissociate into COO^- and H^+. The negative and positive signs indicate that in this dissociation, the hydrogen atom loses its single electron to the combination of one carbon and two oxygen atoms, which is attached to a fourth atom or group of atoms. The hydrogen atom is now a bare proton with a positive charge, the presence of which gives the chemical characteristics of an acid.

Many organic compounds contain more than one oxygen group. For example, pyruvic and lactic acids, both important metabolites (see 'Metabolism'), are respectively an oxoacid (or ketoacid) and a hydroxyacid, the latter being formed by the addition of two hydrogen atoms to the former:

$$\underset{\text{pyruvic acid}}{\begin{array}{c} CH_3 \\ | \\ CO \\ | \\ COOH \end{array}} \xrightarrow{2H} \underset{\text{lactic acid}}{\begin{array}{c} CH_3 \\ | \\ CHOH \\ | \\ COOH \end{array}}$$

When a hydroxyl compound (one containing an OH group) combines with a carboxylic acid (one containing a COOH group), water is eliminated giving an ester, a compound linked by an esteric bond:

$$\underset{\text{ethanol}}{C_2H_5OH} + \underset{\text{acetic acid}}{CH_3 \cdot COOH} \rightleftharpoons \underset{\text{ethyl acetate}}{C_2H_5O \cdot CO\text{-}CH_3} + \underset{\text{water}}{H_2O}$$

The esteric bond in ethyl acetate is here represented by the ($\cdot$) between the atoms $^-O \cdot CO^-$. The two arrows indicate that the reaction can, under suitable conditions, go either way because ethyl acetate (or any other ester) is slowly hydrolysed (that is, split by hydrolysis) in the presence of water.

We return now to our food, and particularly to its fat content. Esters of glycerol, a trihydric alcohol or one which contains three hydroxyl groups, are the major constituents of natural fats and of oils such as olive oil. Each hydroxyl group forms an ester, giving a fat called a triglyceride:

$$\underset{\text{glycerol}}{\begin{array}{c} CH_2OH \\ | \\ CHOH \\ | \\ CH_2OH \end{array}} \qquad \underset{\text{triglyceride}}{\begin{array}{c} CH_2O \cdot CO \cdot R_1 \\ | \\ CH_2O \cdot CO \cdot R_2 \\ | \\ CH_2O \cdot CO \cdot R_3 \end{array}}$$

In this case R indicates a carbon chain, and the use of three different subscripts (1, 2 and 3) indicates that each carbon chain in a single fat molecule may be different.

Starch and sugar are carbohydrates, a word which means 'hydrate of carbon', because they contain hydrogen and oxygen in the same proportion as water (that is, two H to one O). Sugars, for example, have the general formula, $C_nH_{2n}O_n$. They contain either an aldehyde group (CHO) or a keto group (CO) attached to one carbon atom, and hydroxyl groups (OH) attached to each of the others. Thus they can be classified as aldoses or ketoses, and, in addition, according to the number of carbon atoms they contain, as trioses (3C), tetroses (4C), pentoses (5C), hexoses (6C), etc. Among the most common sugars in living organisms are glucose (which is the main blood sugar), an aldohexose, and fructose, its corresponding keto-hexose:

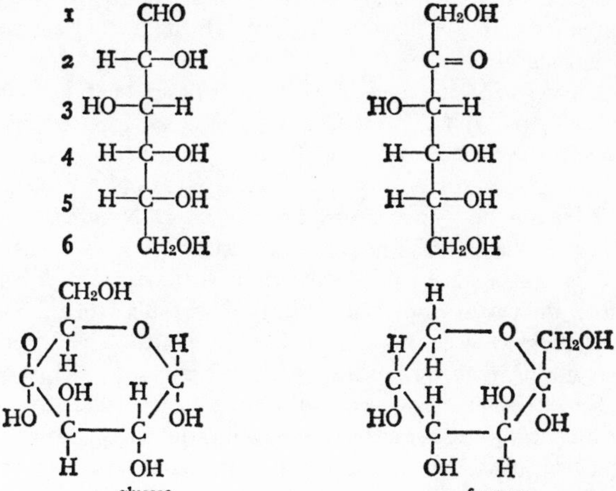

glucose

fructose

Ribose, the sugar moiety of the genetically relevant molecules, deoxyribonucleic acid (DNA) and ribonucleic acid (RNA), is an aldopentose.

The molecules of glucose and fructose shown above are single sugar units, or monosaccharides. They can combine into twos, disaccharides, or into many, polysaccharides. Thus glucose is stored in the liver and muscle of higher animals as a polysaccharide called glycogen.

Proteins are substances in which atoms of nitrogen occur along with carbon, hydrogen, oxygen and, much less frequently, other elements such as sulphur. In proteins, the nitrogen atoms are usually part of the group $-NH_2$; when this group is attached to a hydrocarbon group, the compound is called an amine. For example, $CH_3 \cdot NH_2 =$ methylamine, or

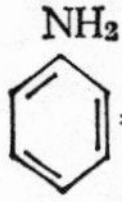

When the $-NH_2$ is attached to a carboxylic acid (one containing a carboxyl group: $-COOH$) rather than directly to a hydrocarbon group, the compound is called an amide; for example, $CH_3-CO-NH_2$, acetamide. The constituents of acetamide (acetic acid, CH_3COOH, and ammonia, NH_3) have combined with the loss of a molecule of water, which was derived partly from the carboxyl group (an O and an H) and partly from the ammonia (an H).

Amino acids, the units of which proteins are built, have an amino group (NH_2) attached to the carbon atom immediately adjacent to the carboxyl group (COOH). They are represented by the general formula, $NH_2-CHR-COOH$, in which R stands for the side chain or ring composed of C, H, O, N and possibly other elements, which make up a particular amino acid. There are in fact about twenty different amino acids (one of them differs from the rest in respect to a structural part other than the R group) which occur in proteins. Different proteins – and there are literally thousands of them in living organisms – consist of long chains of amino acids in various combinations. These chains are formed because amino acids link together by means of peptide bonds; that is, bonds which form between the carboxyl group of one amino acid and the amino group of the next:

$$\underset{R_1}{NH_2 \cdot CH \cdot CO} - NH \underset{R_2}{\cdot CH \cdot CO} - NH \underset{R_3}{\cdot CH \cdot CO} - - - - NH \underset{R_4}{\cdot CH \cdot COOH}$$

↑ peptide bonds ↑

Note that the peptide bonds (CO−NH) are of the amide type. Thus the bonds show chemical properties associated with amides rather than with amines in respect to their cleavage by hydrolysis, for example.

In living organisms, proteins serve two major purposes: those such as collagen, a principal constituent of connective tissue, are structural. Structural proteins, in many instances in combination with other molecules, make up hair, nails, skin, muscle fibres and the membranes of cells and of organelles within cells.

The second major group of proteins are catalytic molecules called enzymes (q.v.). Several antibiotics (q.v.) contain protein molecules, and shorter polypeptide chains (that is, a small number of amino acids connected by peptide bonds) appear in several hormones (q.v.).

To complete this brief summary of certain basic biochemical phenomena, it is necessary to refer once more to the energy which powers organic reactions in lieu of external energy supplies (heat, nuclear fission) obviously not available within living cells. Heat energy derives from the combustion in oxygen of wood or coal, for example; that is, the breakdown of carbohydrates and other substances, and their conversion into carbon dioxide (CO_2) and water. Both of these smaller, simpler molecules require less energy for their creation than did the complex molecules from which they came. By analogy, it is said that the cell 'burns' food to obtain the energy it requires in order to synthesize complex molecules such as proteins. Although the fats, carbohydrates and proteins of food are of course a major source of cellular energy, the image suggested by the word 'burns' is misleading. Combustion converts large molecules directly to CO_2 and H_2O. The cell produces the same end products gradually, almost by the removal of one atom at a time from the complex molecules, though the total process takes place very rapidly.

The energy released by the catabolism (breakdown) of food must be made available for biosynthetic processes in usable packets. These packets are mediated by the electrons which form chemical bonds (just as is energy from all sources in nature); that is, the bonds between atoms represent energy analogous to the much greater energy which holds together the nucleus of atoms and which is released when the atom 'decays' radioactively, or is torn apart in what is called a nuclear explosion. To understand this concept of energy, it must be seen as a measurable event, which means that, for convenience, energy can be broken down, like space is broken down into inches or like weight into ounces. Thus, the energy of a bond between two atoms can be measured in terms of certain features of the electrons which cause the bond to exist because, as negatively charged particles, they are drawn towards the positively charged protons of nearby atomic nuclei. The relevant electronic features might very roughly be described collectively as fields of force, but they can only be defined exactly in the language of mathematics (for which English, or French, or Russian is a poor substitute). It is because electrons, protons and other subatomic particles are at the same time both things (with dimension and weight) and events, that mass and energy can be placed on opposite sides of an equals sign ($=$) in the famous Einsteinian equation: energy equals mass times the speed of light squared. As the cell catabolizes complex molecules, therefore, part of the bond energy from the molecules is transferred to a special kind of energy-storage molecule, adenosine triphosphate (ATP). ATP uniquely performs this vital function in all known life forms.

Adenosine is composed of an amino acid, adenine and of a ribose sugar unit. To the ribose end of the adenosine molecule is attached a chain of three phosphate molecules:

$$\text{adenosine}-O-\underset{\underset{OH}{|}}{\overset{\overset{O}{\|}}{P}}-O-\underset{\underset{OH}{|}}{\overset{\overset{O}{\|}}{P}}-O-\underset{\underset{OH}{|}}{\overset{\overset{O}{\|}}{P}}-OH$$

Certain characteristics of the phosphate bonds, which are esteric bonds analogous to those in triglycerides, require high energy to form them so that equally large amounts of energy are released when they are broken. A very large proportion of all biochemical processes are thus related directly or indirectly to the formation or breakdown of ATP.

Chlorambucil

(Synthesized: J. L. Everett, *et al.*, 1953, U.K.) Trade name: Leukeran. Administration: orally, in tablet form.

Classification
One of a class of drugs known as nitrogen mustards which are closely related to the sulphur mustard used as poison gas during World War I. In the course of research into chemical-warfare possibilities of the nitrogen mustards before and during World War II, it was discovered experimentally that the compounds caused regression of tumours in doses which were tolerated by the host. Other drugs of the same class currently in clinical use are mechloethamine, cyclophosphamide, melphalan, uracil mustard, mustine.

Therapeutic uses
Chlorambucil is the treatment of choice in chronic lymphocytic leukaemia, and has been recommended more recently for ovarian tumours. It may also produce temporary relief of varying duration in Hodgkin's disease, lymphomas, some solid tumours and certain other cancers of blood-element-forming tissues. In

combination with methotrexate (q.v.) and actinomycin D (q.v.), it controls testicular cancers. The drug is thus used for management of a wide range of carcinomas and leukaemias, but it is not considered to be a cure, there being at present very few cures for this extensive group of diseases.

Side effects

Popularly known as tissue-destroying drugs, the nitrogen mustards are effective against rapidly dividing cell populations which occur in many though by no means all types of cancer. Unfortunately, the healthy mammalian body also contains tissues characterized by rapid cell division such as the testicles, or the bone marrow where various kinds of blood cells are formed.

Chlorambucil can cause damage to normal, healthy bone marrow, though fortunately this effect is usually rapidly reversible when the drug is discontinued. Occasionally, other side effects have been noted. They include gastrointestinal discomfort, dermatitis and some liver damage. Excessive doses can cause nausea and vomiting as well as lethargy, convulsions and coma, all due to effects on the brain and spinal cord. Damage to lymph-forming tissue and to the formative cells of the cornea may also occur, and some sterility has been noted due to actions of the drug against sperm-forming cells of the testicles. Nevertheless, chlorambucil is considered to be the least toxic of the nitrogen mustards.

Chemistry and physiology

Like other nitrogen mustards, chlorambucil is an alkylating agent. Its chemical structure is as follows (the portion contained within the dotted box being common to all drugs of the class):

$$HOOC-CH_2-CH_2-CH_2- \text{\textless benzene ring\textgreater} -N \begin{cases} CH_2-CH_2-Cl \\ CH_2-CH_2-Cl \end{cases}$$

Under conditions which exist within both normal body cells and tumour cells, an alkylating agent causes the replacement in an organic molecule of a hydrogen atom, a nitrogen atom, a carboxyl group (COOH; see 'Biochemistry,') or a hydroxyl group (OH) by an alkyl group (CH_2). Such modifications can so alter the organic molecule as to destroy its ability to function normally within the cell. In particular, the nitrogen mustards prevent the correct replication of the gene-carrying deoxyribonucleic acid (DNA) molecule in the nucleus of the cell with the result that daughter cells malfunction and die. The exact method by means of which the compounds act against DNA is not known, though one widely accepted hypothesis holds that one nitrogen atom in one type of base on the DNA molecule (guanine) is alkylated with the result that the two strands of DNA are bound together abnormally at points where this base occurs. In consequence, the strands cannot separate and reproduce themselves accurately during cell division.

Chlorothiazide

(Synthesized: Novello and Sprague, 1957, U.S.) Trade names: Chlotride, Diuril, Saluric. Administration: oral.

Classification
The first clinically useful agent in a class of chemicals called benzothiadiazides, developed during research into improved diuretics, that is, drugs which increase the flow of urine. These chemicals are related to the sulphonamides (q.v.), and include many other drugs: diazoxide, hydrochlorothiazide, benzthiazide, fluomethiazide, trichlormethiazide, polythiazide, etc. Except for special purposes, such as the emergency use of diazoxide ('Therapeutic uses', below), none of them is considered preferable to chlorothiazide.

Therapeutic uses
As a diuretic, the agent is employed to combat oedema, the accumulation of excess intercellular fluid, which may arise from many pathological conditions. Treatment with the drug is usually combined with dietary restrictions on salt intake. Chlorothiazide is indicated for diuresis to reduce oedema caused by chronic heart disease. It is also useful in chronic diseases of the liver or kidney to reduce fluid, but should not be employed when the malfunctions are acute. The benzothiadiazides help in the management of certain pregnancy-related blood disturbances, and in the treatment of pre-menstrual oedema.

Paradoxically, these agents are now also used clinically to treat a disease in which too much urine is excreted. Called diabetes insipidus, the condition is apparently unrelated to diabetes mellitus (see 'Chlorpropamide', 'Insulin') except that its effect is also dehydration and serious disruption of the balance of acids and bases throughout the body. Chlorothiazide and drugs related to it cause only a slight, temporary diuresis in persons with normal or below normal amounts of body fluid. In those with excess fluid excretion, these compounds will effectively decrease the volume of urine after about two days. Salt intake must also be rigorously controlled, however.

More or less by accident, this class of chemicals, and particularly chlorothiazide, were found to have an anti-hypertensive effect. Hypertension describes a variety of conditions, but all of them are characterized by abnormally high constrictive tension of muscle cells in small peripheral blood vessels, especially the arterioles which connect arteries to capillaries. Usually, therefore, hypertension is revealed as high blood pressure which can lead to atherosclerosis and heart disease, kidney malfunctions or failure, cerebral haemorrhage and other extremely serious conditions. Its origins and development are not understood.

The benzothiadiazides are the most widely used agents for the control of mild hypertension, and play a role in the treatment of more severe forms. Excepting diazoxide (which is not a diuretic), however, they are not sufficiently fast or powerful to be used in hypertensive emergencies caused by head injuries or acute kidney or heart failure.

The drug acts slowly and has only a limited effect on blood pressure. Increasing the dosage does not increase the action. For this reason, and because their diuretic action delays excretion of some of these compounds (e.g. mecamylamine and pempidine), chlorothiazide is frequently used in combination with more powerful agents that block sympathetic nervous transmissions (see 'Propranolol', 'Adrenaline', also 'Chemistry and physiology' below).

Side effects
Undesirable effects are rare. Those that do occur result either from allergy-like reactions to the drug, or from the combination of the drug's action and the disease itself. Thus, a weakened kidney can be further damaged by the diuretic effect of the agent. Dermatitis and skin sensitivity to light as well as certain forms of anaemia may occur as a result of allergic reactions. In a few cases, the drug is thought to have caused liver damage. Other side effects can include elevated blood sugar levels which may

lead to diabetes mellitus, gout resulting from the tendency of the drug to retain uric acid in the plasma (i.e. blood without its formed elements; see 'Allopurinol'), and depression.

Chemistry and physiology

Like acetazolamide (q.v.), chlorothiazide inhibits an enzyme (q.v.), carbonic anhydrase, which among other functions is essential for the secretion of electrolytes (q.v.) into the urine by kidney cells. The benzothiadiazides are relatively weak carbonic anhydrase inhibitors, however. Their diuretic action is described as an increase in the excretion of sodium, chloride and water resulting from inhibition of the reabsorption from urine into the bloodstream of sodium and chloride, and the consequent osmotic retention of water in the urine. Such reabsorption is also the function of certain kidney cells (see 'Diuretic' for a more detailed description of kidney function). The biochemical mechanism by means of which this inhibition occurs at the molecular level is unknown, but unlike the carbonic anhydrase inhibitors, this class of chemicals cause diuresis without regard to the acid-base balance of the body fluids or the amount of fluid first filtered out of the bloodstream by the kidney (the glomerular filtrate).

The antidiuretic action of chlorothiazide which makes it effective in the control of diabetes insipidus is also unclear. It is thought to arise from a slight reduction in the volume of glomerular filtrate with a consequent diminution in flow through the kidney tubule which may reduce water reabsorption both in the tubule and in the collecting tube leading to the urethra. This effect could be helped along by another action displayed by the drug: it reduces reabsorption of sodium in the segment of the tubule farthest away from the glomerulus, the distal tubule. Presumably, the antidiuretic effect occurs only when body fluids and, therefore, blood volume are normal or below normal, whereas when oedema exists and blood volume is above normal, more blood circulates through the glomerulus (and the whole kidney) and is subject to filtration.

It was thought at first that the diuretic action of chlorothiazide led directly to its usefulness for the control of hypertension. Oedema would reflect an elevated volume of circulatory fluid (that is, blood), and this excess would require more work by the heart. Diuresis, on the other hand, does tend to reverse these conditions by reducing the volume of circulatory fluid. But the fact is that diazoxide produces anti-hypertensive effects without diuresis. (Diazoxide might be expected to be superior to chlorothiazide for the treatment of hypertension and, as has been noted above, it is used in emergencies. For continuous treatment, however, the agent is too toxic.) Further experimental evidence indicates that the anti-hypertensive usefulness of these agents, although it may be assisted by diuresis, derives from direct action to relax the muscles that regulate the contraction of precapillary vessels of the peripheral circulatory system. The nature of this action is unknown.

Most anti-hypertensive agents block sympathetic nervous impulses (see 'Adrenaline') to the muscles of peripheral blood vessels, but their action is not specific. Depending on what drug is used, the blockade will affect all nerves of a similar type throughout the body. Thus, their side effects can be serious; for example, like the pre-capillary arterioles, the post-capillary vessels which return blood to the veins are maintained in tonus, or a state of semi-rigidity, by muscle cells containing sympathetic alpha-receptors. Drugs such as reserpine which block alpha-receptors so that they cannot receive transmissions from the proximate nerve fibres will, therefore, relax both pre- and post-capillary vessels. Capillaries have no muscle cells in their walls. In consequence, blood return to the heart is less efficient. When a patient treated with an alpha-blocking drug stands erect, his blood pressure may fall precipitously. Chlorothiazide does not block nervous impulses, nor does it relax the post-capillary vessels so that it does not have postural side effects. Its action seems to be restricted to the peripheral circulatory system.

Chlorpromazine

(Charpentier, 1950, Fr.) Trade names: Amargil, Thorazine, Largactil, Megaphen. Administration: oral, injection; for children: syrup or suppositories.

Classification

As much of the research into new pharmaceuticals during the 1940s stemmed from the discovery of the clinical value of penicillin (q.v.), so chlorpromazine is called by some the drug of the fifties. It is one of a class of chemicals called phenothiazine derivatives. Phenothiazine itself was synthesized in the late nineteenth century, but it was not tested clinically until the 1930s. First applications were in the treatment of worms, and as an anti-histamine-like (see 'Tripelennamine') sedative. Related phenothiazine derivatives now in use include promazine, fluphenazine, prochlorperazine, thioridazine and many others.

Therapeutic uses

Chlorpromazine is today the most widely used of all drugs against psychotic states (see 'Imipramine'). It has largely replaced both electro-convulsive and insulin shock therapy and psychosurgery (e.g. prefrontal lobotomy), as well as other physical treatments such as water and occupational therapy in psychotic disorders. It has been estimated that one per cent of the total population suffers from psychotic disorders which require, though they do not always receive, hospitalization. Until the advent of chlorpromazine, furthermore, mental institutions were frequently prisons rather than hospitals because of a pervasive nihilism among therapists as to the probable efficacy of any treatment. This agent has proved to be effective against paranoia, delusions, social withdrawal and other schizophrenic symptoms, often accompanied by violently destructive behaviour, as well as against milder neurotic states of anxiety and agitation. It is not yet clear that treatment with the drug can be permanently stopped without a return of some symptoms, although about a third of patients have had the compound withdrawn without serious regression. In any event, the condition of most patients after administration is such as to permit a return to home or work even though they may continue to receive the drug.

Chlorpromazine was introduced, and is still employed, for the purpose of preventing vomiting associated with uraemia, gastroenteritis, pregnancy, some effects of cancer, radiation sickness and the use of certain drugs. It can control excessive hiccoughing, a use which has been especially valuable when hiccoughing occurs during surgery.

Side effects

Although neither chlorpromazine nor its related compounds create euphoria or cause addiction in the common sense of the word (physical dependence may exist in relation to the treatment of psychosis, as explained above), it has a wide range of possible side effects. This is scarcely surprising in a drug which acts so powerfully on most of the nervous system. Yet the incidence of side effects appears to be as low as three per cent among the very large number of patients who have received the drug. Its use is, however, almost invariably accompanied by a sedative effect which may occur as a result of the depression of brain centres related to psychotic behaviour. A fall in blood pressure, which may result from actions on the heart, blood vessels and the peripheral nervous system as well as the brain, can be serious in older people, and may cause fainting regardless of age. Somewhat more dangerous, though less frequent, are allergy-like hypersensitivity reactions including abnormal conditions of the blood, obstructive jaundice and skin eruptions. Hypersensitivity reactions occur when the body responds strongly to foreign invasive substances. Chlorpromazine may also cause motor disturbances such as those characteristic of parkinsonism, although it does not appear to depress the higher powers of reasoning even in the presence of such reactions. In some cases, the drug appears to have brought on epileptic seizures. Palpitation, nasal constriction, dryness of the mouth and slight constipation may result from taking the drug. In its presence, barbiturates (see 'Phenobarbitone') work for longer periods, alcohol (see 'Ethyl alcohol') makes the user more inebriated and other drugs such as morphine display stronger effects than is usual.

Chemistry and physiology

The phenothiazines all have the same central molecular structure:

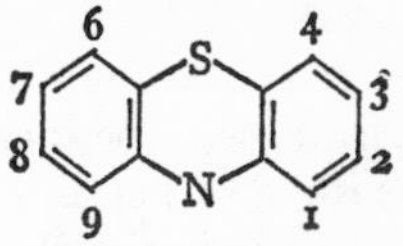

At both the N atom and the carbon atom numbered 2, different atoms or groups of atoms are linked to the central structure. It is these which appear to give the drugs their effects. Thus, chlorpromazine has a chlorine atom attached at the 2 position, and a side chain at the nitrogen atom, as follows: $-CH_2-CH_2-CH_2-N(CH_3)_2$. Though it is known that variations in the attached atoms cause distinctive changes in the effects of the various compounds, their cellular mechanisms of action are unknown. The drugs affect the brain directly, as well as the autonomic nervous system (see 'Adrenaline'), but the physical locations of these effects are complex. In several specific instances, they are also the subject of considerable scientific disagreement. (For discussion of anxiety, see 'Tranquillizer'. For discussion of depression, see 'Imipramine'.

Chlorpropamide

(Marshal and Sigal, 1957, U.S.) Trade name: Diabinase.
Administration: oral.

Classification

Chlorpropamide is a synthetic, one of a class of chemicals called sulphonylureas, related to the sulphonamides (q.v.) from which they were developed. The only other clinically useful drug of this class is an earlier discovery, tolbutamide (trade name: Orinase).

Therapeutic uses

Chlorpropamide is an oral hypoglycaemic: that is, it is administered orally, and lowers the amount of sugar in the blood. It has this action, however, only if blood-sugar content is abnormally high (if the patient is hyperglycaemic). The drug is a treatment for diabetes mellitus, particularly for the form of the disease which occurs after the age of forty and not before the age of thirty (see description of diabetes mellitus under 'Insulin'). It is usually given to patients whose daily insulin requirement has been low; under these conditions, chlorpropamide may substitute entirely for insulin therapy, excepting during fever, surgery or trauma when more sugar is required by tissues.

Chlorpropamide remains in the bloodstream about seven times as long as tolbutamide, and may therefore be given in smaller doses. However, tolbutamide is customarily given first while chlorpropamide is withheld unless the former agent does not produce the desired reduction in blood-sugar level. Other oral hypoglycaemics called biguanides are also used for the treatment of diabetes mellitus, the most satisfactory being phenformin.

Side effects

Chlorpropamide has a very low incidence of undesirable side effects. These can include disturbances of the balance of the formed elements in the blood (e.g. red blood cells, leucocytes), gastrointestinal upset and loss of appetite, and jaundice. Tolbutamide has been subjected to continuing clinical tests because of reported cardiovascular side effects, but it is still considered safe for use when diet alone will not control the disease. Patients receiving either drug may be intolerant of alcohol.

Chemistry and physiology

The biochemical events by means of which the sulphonylureas (a sulphonamide linked to a urea moiety) perform their therapeutic action are unknown. The action itself occurs in the pancreas, however; there, the agents stimulate secretion of insulin (q.v.; see description of pancreas under 'Hormone').

Cholestyramine

(D. M. Tennant, *et al.*, 1965, U.S.) Trade names: Cuemid, Questran. Administration: oral.

Classification
A synthetic drug related to the natural steroid (see 'Hormone'), cholesterol, it also contains the organic compound, tyramine. It derives from a resin or plastic required for the manufacture of an antibiotic (q.v.); its clinical usefulness emerged as a by-product when certain resins were found to reduce reabsorption of liver bile and the absorption of dietary fats from the intestine into the bloodstream.

Therapeutic uses
The first and still the principal use of cholestyramine is for the relief of very severe itching which accompanies an uncommon form of liver disease, primary biliary cirrhosis. In this condition, the cause of which is unknown, the ducts which conduct bile formed in the liver to the upper part of the small intestine are partially blocked. Bile therefore enters the bloodstream in unusually large amounts, and is deposited in various tissues, including the skin, where it causes itching so persistent and serious that it can lead patients to consider suicide.

Cholestyramine also reduces the diarrhoea which may occur after certain intestinal operations, and may help in the control of a less common form of anaemia caused by malfunctions in the biosynthesis of the haem molecule, that portion of the red blood cell which carries oxygen and carbon dioxide. The reason for the usefulness of the compound in this context is unclear.

Potentially, the most important use of the drug is for the treatment of atherosclerosis, the common condition popularly known as hardening of the arteries. Cholestyramine reduces the absorption of food fats and contributes to a reduction in blood cholesterol which is thought to be a cause of atherosclerosis, though not the only one. Clinical trials of the drug for treatment of this condition are under way.

Side effects

Because cholestyramine is not absorbed into the body through the walls of the intestine, side effects are usually mild. Nausea, heartburn, constipation or diarrhoea may occur in the early stages of treatment. Severe diarrhoea with much loss of food fats can follow. Vitamins A, D, E and K (see 'Vitamin') are fat soluble, and if fat absorption is impaired, intake of these vitamins may be inadequate, requiring supplemental injections to maintain the requisite amounts in the body. A mild acidification of the body fluids may occur with high doses, and, in a few cases, the drug may have contributed to formation of gallstones. Perhaps the most immediate side effect is an extremely unpleasant odour of bad fish when the drug is taken. The newer preparation, Questran, is more palatable.

Chemistry and physiology

The agent is an insoluble chloride salt (a chemical combination of an acid and a base with the loss of water). In this case, the acidic constituent is chloride. Cholestyramine acts in the intestine where it gives up chloride leaving a basic molecule which binds with bile acid to form a bile salt, a cholate. The resultant complex is insoluble and is excreted in the faeces. It is for this reason that the agent never enters body cells, fluids or intercellular spaces, but remains on the surface, so to speak ('Side effects', above).

Bile is principally employed to aid the absorption of fat particles through the intestinal walls. The mechanisms of fat absorption are in fact not fully understood, but the process begins with the enzymic (see 'Enzyme') breakdown of fat particles from food into fatty acid and other fat-like molecules, some of which are soluble in water while others are not. The former can enter directly into the cells of the intestinal wall which then pass them out, often metabolically altered, partly into the capillaries but chiefly into the tiny lymphatics near by. These vessels carry tissue fluid (lymph), absorbed fat and foreign materials which have been introduced into the tissues, back to the bloodstream. They function as a drainage and filtering system rather than as a circulatory system (and do not contain blood). The insoluble particles of fat are thought to combine with the bile in which form they too can enter cells of the intestinal wall. Thus, the constituents of bile re-enter the body along with the water-insoluble food-fat particles.

Bile itself is synthesized in the liver from cholesterol plus other substances, and major precursors of cholesterol (which is also synthesized within the body) derive from food fats. When cholestyramine inhibits reabsorption of bile, therefore, it has a double effect. First, it interferes with the normal absorption of dietary fats which are excreted instead. Second, it forces the body to draw on existing supplies of bile precursors, especially cholesterol, so that the supply of bile can be maintained.

The drug prevents the itching of primary biliary cirrhosis apparently because it forces a reduction in the amount of bile carried by the blood. If the bile ducts are completely blocked, however, the itching is not reduced by the drug. When the compound is withdrawn, furthermore, itching will in most cases recur.

Although some advantage may be derived from reduction in the absorption of food fats, the potential usefulness of cholestyramine for the treatment of atherosclerosis is assumed to arise principally from its second effect, above: reduction in cholesterol supplies. In fact, the current clinical trials are testing two related questions: first and foremost, is a high plasma level of cholesterol a cause of atherosclerosis so that a reduction in the level of the sterol reduces the incidence of the condition? Second, is the body able to compensate for decreased stores of cholesterol by increased biosynthesis of the steroid? In other words, if cholesterol content falls below a certain point, will not compensatory mechanisms stimulate some alternative metabolic pathways, the use of which is not normally required for the formation of cholesterol?

Cocaine

(Clinical use: S. Freud and K. Köller, 1884, Aust.)
Administration: topical.

Classification
Cocaine was the first local anaesthetic. It derives from an Andean shrub, *Erythroxylon coca*, the leaves of which are chewed by the *alta plana* Indians of Ecuador and Peru because they give a sense of well-being. Although ethyl alcohol (q.v.) has anaesthetic properties when it is injected, the commonly used local anaesthetics are synthetic compounds. The oldest, procaine (Novocain), is still the most widely used. Lidocaine (Xylocaine) acts more rapidly and lasts longer than procaine, but it is also more toxic. Both of these synthetic drugs may be injected as well as employed topically.

Therapeutic uses

The local anaesthetics may be used whenever pain exists or is anticipated but a general anaesthetic (see 'Halothane') is either undesirable or impractical. These circumstances include treatment of wounds, dentistry, ophthalmology, childbirth, and even the control of chronic pain over long periods, though local anaesthetics employed for chronic pain may cause tissue damage.

Cocaine has been largely displaced from clinical practice by the synthetics. In the manner of Sherlock Holmes, cocaine is used today illegally as a stimulant, for which purpose the drug is inhaled as a powder, but it may be of clinical value for a patient who has displayed an allergic reaction to the synthetic agents. None of the synthetics possesses the power to stimulate the brain cortex as does cocaine.

Side effects

Unlike the synthetic local anaesthetics, cocaine is a drug of addiction. Tolerance develops to its stimulatory effects, and withdrawal produces various symptoms. Acute cocaine poisoning can be rapidly fatal. The patient becomes excited and then anxious. Headache, nausea and vomiting are common. A chill develops, quickly followed by fever. Touch hallucinations may occur. Delirium, breathing difficulties, convulsions and coma are followed by death due to respiratory collapse. In some cases, the patient collapses and dies almost immediately after using cocaine, probably because the drug impairs heart action directly. The best treatment for acute cocaine poisoning is injection of a short-acting barbiturate (see 'Phenobarbitone') to counteract the central nervous depression that produces respiratory collapse. Artificial respiration may also be necessary.

The use of cocaine in the eye greatly enlarges the pupil. It may also cause damage to the cornea, a side effect not produced by the synthetic drugs.

Procaine is about one quarter as toxic as cocaine and rarely causes poisoning. However, one of its breakdown products is para-aminobenzoic acid, the substance with which the sulphonamides (q.v.) compete in order to halt the growth of bacteria. Procaine and many similar synthetic compounds cannot be used if the patient is taking a sulphonamide.

Cocaine is chemically similar to the synthetics though its molecule is somewhat more complex. The mechanism of action of none of the agents is known, but they all prevent the generation and block the conduction of nerve impulses. They seem to alter characteristics of the nerve cell membrane so that the movement of ions (q.v.) through the membrane changes from the normal. Inasmuch as the nerve impulse reflects ionic flows into and out of nerve cells, any change in the properties of nerve cell membranes might be expected to change cellular functions.

In general, small nerve cells are more responsive to local anaesthetics than larger cells. All of the senses are affected by the drugs, but pain is the first to disappear. The synthetic compounds affect the brain, but they are not addictive because they are much less stimulatory at the cortex.

Unlike the synthetics, cocaine causes constriction of blood vessels. This action appears to be due to the effect of the drug on the brain. The reduced blood flow slows the dissipation of the drug from the site of application and prolongs its anaesthetic action. This is a desirable quality in a local anaesthetic, and to achieve the same end with the synthetics, they may be administered with a low dose of adrenaline (q.v.) or a similar drug.

Dicoumarol. U.S.: Bishydroxycoumarin

(Link, 1943–4, U.S.) Trade name: none. Administration: oral.

Classification

One of a class of drugs called coumarins which were isolated from spoiled sweet clover. It had been noted that the rotted forage caused fatal haemorrhages in cattle which ate it (Schofield, 1922–4, U.S.). Related agents include ethyl biscoumacetate, warfarin, phenprocoumon, acenocoumarin and cyclocoumarol. Another, chemically unrelated group of drugs called diones, and including phenindione, diphenadione and anisindione, have therapeutic uses similar to those of the coumarins. Both the coumarins and the diones are synthetic compounds.

Therapeutic uses

All of these drugs are called oral anti-coagulants because they are used for the prevention of unwanted blood clotting. Their uses are similar to those of heparin (q.v.), and that entry should be read with this one. Because heparin must be injected, dicoumarol and related drugs have the advantage for long courses of treatment. Heparin is also more expensive, but it acts almost immediately upon injection, whereas the oral anti-coagulants take up to twenty-four hours to exert their effect. Heparin is often used at the beginning of a course of treatment, and the oral drug for its continuation. Dicoumarol and the other oral drugs have a much longer period of action than heparin with peak effects remaining up to four days. Thus, if an unwanted side effect should appear, it is harder to be rid of it with dicoumarol than with heparin.

Side effects

Neither dicoumarol nor the other anti-coagulants should be administered during pregnancy, or in the presence of ulcers, liver diseases, certain cardiovascular disorders, surgically in-duced kidney malfunctions, pre-existing bleeding tendencies (e.g. haemophilia), or cerebrospinal accidents (e.g. a stroke) unless the cause is recent surgery or trauma such as a blow to the head. Long-term treatment with these drugs is also unwise if the patient suffers from chronic alcoholism or is undergoing intensive treatment with aspirin (q.v.) or a related drug.

Although untoward effects are rare, dicoumarol can cause gastrointestinal disturbances. Warfarin has occasionally pro-duced loss of hair, dermatitis and hives, while phenindione has caused blood disorders, hepatitis and jaundice. As with heparin, the most serious side effect of any of these agents can be haemor-rhage. Avoidance of bleeding on the one hand, and of throm-bosis (that is, blockage of a blood vessel by a blood clot inside it) on the other, requires maintenance of a delicate balance between the clotting factors (see 'Heparin') and the natural anti-coagulants in the blood, probably including heparin. Individual variation in response to the anti-coagulants is very great. A patient receiving any of these drugs must obviously remain under the most careful observation.

Chemistry and physiology

The mechanism of action of dicoumarol is unknown. It appears to be an anti-metabolite (see 'Metabolism'), of vitamin K, and the effects of the drug can be offset by the vitamin (q.v.). Intravenous injection of vitamin K, furthermore, is essential to halt haemorrhaging which arises from use of any anti-coagulant.

The oral compounds block the synthesis by liver cells of certain substances required for the formation of a blood clot: prothrombin and factors VII, IX and X, at least two of which (factors VII and IX) may be derived from prothrombin. All four substances are required for the biosynthesis of thromboplastin.

The drugs thus indirectly inhibit prothrombin formation. (For further details of the complex processes required for blood clotting, see 'Heparin'.)

Digitalis

(Withering, 1785, Eng.; ascription of heart action: Ferrier, 1799, Eng.) Trade names: as common chemical names. Administration: oral or, if necessary, by injection.

Classification
A clinically useful mixture of three drugs derived from either of two plants: digitoxin and gitoxin occur naturally in the leaves of *Digitalis purpurea* (foxglove) and of *Digitalis lanata*. Gitalin is a constituent of the former, and digoxin, of the latter. Drugs with almost identical therapeutic uses derive from the seeds of *Strophanthus* (ouabain and cymarin) and from squill, the bulb of the sea onion, *Urginea maritima* (proscillaridin A). All of these agents are known as cardiac glycosides.

Therapeutic uses
By far the most important therapeutic use of digitalis is in the treatment of congestive heart failure. In this condition, the heart is persistently unable to maintain blood circulation adequate for tissue needs for oxygen and nutrients. Death usually ensues from total heart collapse, rather than from gradual anoxia (oxygen lack). Digitalis reverses the symptoms – oedema (see 'Diuretic'), enlargement of the heart, breathlessness and decreased blood volume, among others – and controls the condition itself, but it is not a cure. Most patients given digitalis for congestive heart failure must continue to receive it for the rest of their lives.

The heart is of course a pump, the functions of which are to circulate the blood for oxygenation (in the lungs), to provide nutrition (to all tissues), to allow oxygen–carbon dioxide exchange (between tissue and blood, and blood and lungs), and removal of wastes (from tissue through kidneys, lungs and skin), as well as for a myriad of less superficially obvious physiological purposes. Blood enters the right atrium (see diagram) from the great veins, the inferior and superior venae cavae. At the beginning of systole (contraction), the right atrium empties blood into the right ventricle, from which it is ejected into the pulmonary artery. During diastole (relaxation), blood returns through the pulmonary vein to the left atrium, from which it enters the left ventricle at the beginning of the next systole. The fourth compartment, the left ventricle, is much the most heavily muscled, and pumps blood into the aorta for general circulation, as well as into the coronary artery to meet the requirements of the heart itself.

In the normal heart, the heartbeat originates with specialized pacemaker cells at the sinu-atrial (SAN) node in the upper rear wall of the right atrium. The contraction of these cells establishes an impulse which spreads to adjacent muscle cells in expanding circles like ripples on the surface of a pond, until they reach the atrio-ventricular (AVN) node. This second specialized group of heart-muscle cells, located in the wall separating right and left atria just above the valves which separate the atria from the ventricles, reinforces the impulse in a manner analogous to a booster power station, and transmits it along additional highly conductive tissue into the muscle of the ventricles. Although these nodes, and the muscle cells, are regulated by the autonomic nervous system (see 'Adrenaline', 'Atropine', also 'Chemistry and physiology' below), they can contract independently of nervous stimulation. Analogously, the ventricles can contract independently of the atria (or, in pathological conditions, of each other). It is for this reason that digitalis therapy can be aimed at the ventricles, the essential pumping stations, even when atrial malfunctions may apparently be increased by the drug.

If heart failure is brought on by hypertension or atherosclerosis (see 'Chlorothiazide' 'Methyldopa'), digitalis promises the best results. The agent may also be used when the cause of failure is infection, anaemia or thyroid malfunction, but in such cases, it is very important to treat the underlying condition as well. On the whole, the failing heart will respond to cardiac glycosides if it possesses any reserve heart muscle strength, but not if it has been too badly damaged as a result of the causative

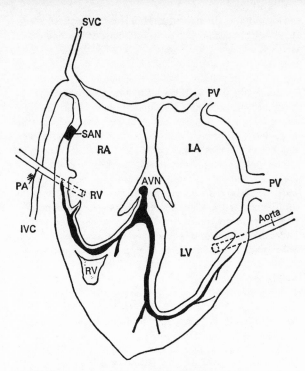

Diagram of section through mammalian heart

SVC = Superior vena cava	RV = Right ventricle
IVC = Inferior vena cava	LA = Left atrium
PA = Pulmonary artery	LV = Left ventricle
SAN = Sinu-atrial node	AVN = Atrio-ventricular node
RA = Right atrium	PV = Pulmonary vein

The black lines running down through the heart wall separating the ventricles (the intraventricular septum) represent specialized muscle cells which conduct nervous impulses from the atrio-ventricular node. The pulmonary artery and aorta are added to the diagram to show the chambers from which they arise, but would not appear in a section of the heart along this plane.

Adapted from George H. Bell, J. N. Davidson and H. Scarborough, *Textbook of Physiology and Biochemistry*, Edinburgh and London, 1968, p. 544.

malfunction. Some physicians recommend digitalis for prophylactic treatment of patients with cardiovascular disease to prevent the signs of heart failure. Only the toxicity of the agent ('Side effects', below) appears to limit its usefulness as a preventive.

Use of the drug is also indicated in certain other heart conditions: atrial fibrillation exists when the muscle fibres of the atria no longer respond to the impulse originated by the S-A node (or the node may cease to provide an impulse) so that the atria contract arrhythmically; that is, each fibre acts more or less independently of its neighbour. Atrial flutter is an arrhythmia which may occur prior to fibrillation. In both conditions, digitalis can maintain an adequate output from the right ventricle to the lungs, and from the left ventricle to the general circulation and to the heart muscle itself. Paroxysmal tachycardia, an erratic speeding up of heart action, may also be controlled by the drug if it occurs in the atria or in the A-V node, but not if the tachycardia occurs in the ventricles where digitalis treatment may be dangerous. Coronary thrombosis and angina pectoris (see 'Dicoumarol', 'Heparin') do not respond to cardiac glycosides, but one of this class of drugs is nevertheless used if either condition appears to be accompanied by heart failure.

Side effects
In large doses, or after the cumulative effects of long-term treatment, digitalis and all other cardiac glycosides can produce fatal intoxication. Because of differences of reaction among patients, and because of the respect accorded to digitalis preparations by physicians, with the resultant care in their use, the lethal dose of the drug is unknown. Symptoms of digitalis poisoning may include loss of appetite, nausea, vomiting, diarrhoea, abdominal pain, and increase in heart arrhythmias leading to atrial and ventricular fibrillation (the latter being the most frequent cause of death), headache, fatigue, drowsiness, delirium, and vision disturbances. Skin rashes and other reactions occur rarely, and in a few men, the drug appears to induce the growth of breast tissue, possibly because it is chemically related to female hormones (q.v.; see also: 'Oestradiol', 'Progesterone'; also 'Chemistry and physiology', below) – although it is no less closely related to male hormone (see 'Testosterone').

Digitalis poisoning can be stopped by withdrawal of the drug, and possibly by treatment with potassium, providing heart malfunctions arising from it have not progressed too far. Propranolol (q.v.) can also be useful.

Although all cardiac glycosides have similar therapeutic effects, they differ in the length of time required for their actions to start, and in duration. Digitalis and digitoxin have the slowest time of onset (twenty-five minutes to two hours) and the longest period of duration (two to three weeks); ouabain is at the other extreme (three to ten minutes, and one to three days, respectively).

Chemistry and physiology

In addition to the natural glycosides ('Classification', above), several semi-synthetic compounds have been produced, but only one of them, acetyldigoxin, is used clinically. All drugs in this class contain a steroid structure (see 'Hormone') to the A ring of which is attached one or more sugar molecules (thus the term glyco-side); to the D ring, an unsaturated ring (see 'Biochemistry') is attached. The steroid nucleus plus the unsaturated ring is called an aglycone or genin. Although the aglycone is known to be the active portion of the molecule, the molecular mechanism of action is unclear.

The drug molecule may act partly on the A–V node cells altering their degree of excitability, and partly by altering the balance of the regulatory activities of the two divisions of the autonomic system (see 'Adrenaline', and below). It has been shown that the drug alters the permeability of the cell membrane to certain electrolytes (q.v.), especially calcium ions. It is also possible that the agent potentiates an enzyme (q.v.), sodium-and-potassium-stimulated adenosine triphosphatase, which is concerned with the supply of energy required to allow the interlinked transportation of sodium and potassium across cell membranes. This movement of electrolytes into and out of the cell is essential to the activity both of muscle and of nerves. The toxic effects of digitalis overdosage, furthermore, appear to be related to inhibition of the enzyme, and potassium acts as an antidote because the ions cause some of the drug molecules to be released from cell receptors that mediate inhibition.

Thus, the drug is thought possibly to act directly on heart muscle as well as on the nerves which regulate the organ. Increased activity of the vagus nerve, part of the parasympathetic system (see 'Atropine'), exerts a damping effect on ventricular action by an effect on the atria which alters conduction through the A–V node, whereas the sympathetic innervation is excitatory. In general, it seems that therapeutic doses of the cardiac glycosides increase the influence of the vagus nerve and reduce sympathetic activity. Higher toxic doses, however, may have the opposite effect, and indeed so excite the sympathetic fibres that fibrillation can occur.

In contrast to the molecular mechanism of action, the gross pharmacological effect of these drugs is fairly well understood, given that heart action is for good reason subject to perhaps the most complex interrelated controls in the body. Digitalis increases the amplitude of the heartbeat, not the rate but the 'size' and regularity of the stroke.

In all subjects, autonomic nervous stimulation, as well as the secretion of some hormones (q.v.) relevant to heart action, is regulated in part by brain centres which receive sensory data with respect to the heart from pressure receptors (sensitive to changes in blood pressure) and chemical receptors (sensitive to changes in the oxygen–carbon dioxide content, or more precisely, the resultant acid-base content of the blood). By increasing heart stroke, digitalis increases the amount of blood being oxygenated by the lungs as well as the pressure of blood in the general circulation. In the normal heart, these effects set up nervous reflexes which tend to contradict the drug action, and this may explain the lack of effect of digitalis in normal subjects. These considerations do not apparently apply to the heart approaching failure, however.

Improved respiratory circulation tends to correct the breathlessness and other disturbances of oxygenation which accompany heart failure. By altering the acid-base and electrolyte (q.v.) content of the blood, it contributes indirectly to the mobilization of oedematous fluid, though this improvement is also a result of better general circulation. In other words, diuresis occurs for several reasons. The enhanced sense of well-being resulting from more normal heart action may lead to a better appetite (a result also of more normal blood oxygenation and acid-base balance), which in turn increases the blood content through protein extracted from food. This 'richer' blood tends to cause tissue fluids to enter blood vessels to a greater extent, due to the simple physical process of osmosis. The increased rate of pumping by the heart decreases the pressure in the veins, and restores normal pressure differentials between small arteries, from which fluid first enters tissues, and small veins through which it returns to the blood so that hydrodynamic tissue drainage returns towards normal. Finally, the greater volume of circulating blood as well as its altered acid-base content improves kidney function. Indeed, the most obvious early effect of digitalis therapy is diuresis, which explains why Withering considered it a treatment for dropsy (oedematous swelling and weakness) rather than for heart failure, although the English physician did note the connexion between the two.

Dipyridamole

(Basic compound: F. G. Fischer and J. Roch, 1951, Ger.) Trade names: Persantin, Sedapersantin. Administration: oral (intravenous injection for experimental purposes).

Classification, therapeutic use and side effects
Angina pectoris is an acute, extremely painful heart 'seizure' which occurs because of an inadequate supply of oxygen (hypoxia) or of nutrients (ischaemia) to heart muscle (myocardial) cells (see 'Heparin'). Anginal attacks are most often

caused by atherosclerosis (or 'hardening') of the coronary blood vessels. For more than a century, anginal episodes have been treated with nitrites, particularly with glyceryl trinitrate, perhaps better known as nitroglycerin. These useful drugs have three disadvantages, however: they can be poisonous; after continued use, they cease to prevent or to halt an anginal attack; and they do not provide long-term protection against attacks. Dipyridamole was developed as part of the effort to meet these difficulties.

It has been assumed that hypoxia and ischaemia in the myocardium, or in any other tissue, could be prevented if the blood vessels could be kept as wide open as possible, so to speak. Thus the nitrites are vasodilators, as is dipyridamole. Although the latter agent can also halt anginal attacks, whether or not it will prevent them in a statistically significant number of patients is uncertain on present evidence. However, dipyridamole appears to be practically non-toxic, although nausea, diarrhoea, headache and dizziness may occur occasionally after use of the drug. In addition to its short-term effectiveness against angina, which is no greater than that of nitroglycerin, dipyridamole appears also to inhibit the clumping of blood platelets, formed elements in the blood which are involved in the process of clotting, thus reducing the danger of thrombosis. The compound may also be useful in the treatment of conditions in which the heart fails to maintain adequate circulation (see 'Digitalis').

Chemistry and physiology

Dipyridamole is chemically dissimilar from other vasodilators, containing what is called a pyrimido-pyrimidine ring system:

The dotted line encloses a pyrimidine nucleus.

The mechanism of action is unknown, although there is some evidence that the agent retards the metabolic breakdown of nucleotides. These are segments of deoxyribonucleic acid (DNA) and ribonucleic acid (RNA) molecules, and of certain coenzymes (see 'Enzyme', 'Vitamin'); each nucleotide contains a pyrimidine or a purine plus a sugar (ribose) and a phosphate. It is supposed that retardation of catabolism (see 'Metabolism') increases the number of nucleotides in myocardial cells, particularly the number of molecules of certain coenzymes required in the biochemical reactions by means of which cells obtain energy. Thus, in theory the metabolic ability of the heart muscle cells would be enhanced by the drug.

Disulfiram

(Therapeutic use: Hald and Jacobsen, 1948, Denmark) 'Disulfiram' is a trade name for tetraethylthiuram disulphide. Other trade names: Antabuse, Aversan, Abstinyl, Refusal. Administration: oral.

Classification
The compound was originally developed for use in the rubber industry where it was discovered that workers exposed to it developed a hypersensitivity to ethyl alcohol (q.v.).

Therapeutic use
The only clinical use for this drug is in the treatment of chronic alcoholism. It is not a 'cure', however, inasmuch as alcoholism, like the compulsive use of barbiturates (see 'Phenobarbitone') or other narcotics, probably stems from personality problems or mental disturbances for which neither cause nor cure are yet clear.

Side effects
It is of course the very unpleasantness of its actions in the presence of alcohol which gives Disulfiram its value in the treatment of chronic alcoholism. The fact that in extreme cases, use of the drug can be life threatening, however, has led to a search for other agents with similar therapeutic effects. Citrated calcium carbimide and a class of compounds called sulphonylureas, developed as oral antidiabetics (see 'Chlorpropamide'), have been tried with some success. More recently, recognition by doctors that the social and psychological causes of alcoholism

must be dealt with if the patient is not to return to the bottle after treatment, has led to a reduction in the clinical emphasis on chemotherapy.

Possible side effects of Disulfiram in the absence of alcohol can include skin eruptions, allergy-type reactions, fatigue, loss of sexual potency, headache and dizziness, all of them temporary.

Chemistry and physiology

Disulfiram combines chemically with certain metals, especially iron and copper. The connexion, if any, between this action and its biochemical behaviour is not clear, however.

Ethyl alcohol is initially oxidized (see 'Biochemistry') in the body to acetaldehyde by the enzyme (q.v.), alcohol dehydrogenase. Further oxidation then occurs, probably in the main through the action of a second enzyme, aldehyde dehydrogenase, which requires as a coenzyme, nicotinamide adenine dinucleotide (NAD; see also 'Vitamin'). Disulfiram seems to compete with NAD, and to replace the coenzyme at the active chemical centre of aldehyde dehydrogenase, causing the enzyme to lose its ability to catalyse the oxidation of acetaldehyde. This may be its mechanism of action.

Ingestion of even minute amounts of alcohol (one or two teaspoonsful) after drug treatment rapidly builds up the amount of acetaldehyde in the body, and within five to ten minutes produces an acetaldehyde syndrome. At first the face feels hot and then flushes. As the causative dilation of peripheral blood vessels spreads, the whole body flushes, and a throbbing headache may develop. Breathing difficulties, nausea, vomiting, chest pain, a fall in blood pressure upon standing, psychological disturbances, dizziness and blurred vision may ensue. In an extreme reaction, a heart attack, heart failure and death can occur. It is this danger which has limited the use of the drug.

Diuretic (Anti-diuretic)

An agent which increases the secretion of urine. (Thus antidiuretic: one which maintains normal urine volume or reduces urine volume.)

Diuretics are classifiable according to their mechanism of action under two broad headings: those which alter the content of solids in the body fluids, and those which alter the normal functions of the kidney. The former include water, sodium chloride (salt), mannitol (a kind of sugar), urea and ammonium nitrate, but they are less frequently used than diuretics of the second type. These include organic mercurials such as calomel (mercurous oxide) and merbaphen, acetazolamide (q.v.), chlorothiazide (q.v.) and other benzothiadiazides, spironolactone which antagonizes aldosterone, a hormone (q.v.) that reduces kidney water loss, and two newer agents, ethacrynic acid and triamterene.

With the exception of water, all of these agents are employed primarily to treat oedema, an excess of body fluid. This excess, largely water, is outside the cells in intercellular spaces and noncellular connective tissue; although blood volume may also be above normal, oedematous fluid is 'stagnant' rather than circulating. Naturally, therefore, it may cause swelling, the so-called 'dropsical swelling' of heart disease, for example.

There is constant interchange between blood plasma and non-circulating body fluids through the smaller blood vessels. Because the blood in arterioles and capillaries normally retains higher pressure than that in the surrounding body fluids, fluid moves out of the circulation into the intercellular spaces; in the venules, this hydrostatic balance is reversed, as is the normal fluid flow. Thus, if blood pressure is too high, oedema may form because more fluid tends to leave the circulation than to enter it. Organic malfunctions other than high blood pressure can cause oedema, but the overall effects of the condition are similar: swelling and pressure on organs such as the heart, lungs and brain which can damage the tissues. It is almost always desirable, therefore, to enable the body to mobilize and excrete oedematous fluid, and this is accomplished by increasing the urine flow.

The mechanisms of action and side effects of each diuretic drug are distinctive. They are, therefore, selected for use, alone or in combinations, in accordance with the causes and precise nature of the oedematous state, the condition of the patient and the experience and preferences of the physician. It is impossible in the space available to discuss each of them, but they all work via the kidneys.

The mammalian kidney consists of millions of complex tubules (see diagram) held together by connective tissue, with suitable nervous connexions and elaborate blood supplies. At the top or outer end of each tubule is a sac-like structure called a glomerulus in which is a tiny bundle of thin capillaries. Because the pressure of blood inside the capillaries is greater than that of the fluid outside (it is being drained away constantly to form urine),

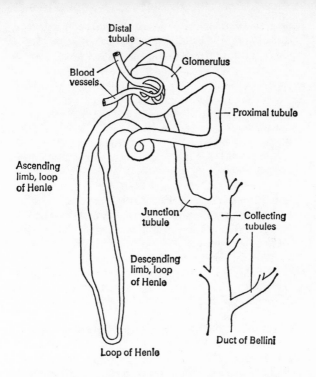

Diagram of single kidney tubule.

Based on George H. Bell, J. N. Davidson, H. Scarborough, *Textbook of Physiology and Biochemistry*, Edinburgh and London, 1968, p. 700.

water, various molecules and electrolytes (q.v.) are filtered through the capillary walls into the glomerulus. So efficient and so numerous are the glomeruli that in a hundred minutes they could effectively remove all fluid from the normal human body. Obviously, most of the material filtered out of the blood by the glomerulus must be returned to it. Reabsorption of about ninety-nine per cent of the glomerular filtrate is the function of the balance of the renal (kidney) tubule. The remaining one per cent passes from the tubule into collecting tubes as urine, although water may also be reabsorbed from the smaller collecting tubes proximate to the tubules.

The renal tubule does not reabsorb filtered components in

exactly the same proportion as they passed from the blood into the glomerulus. In addition to its excretory functions, the kidney is one of the delicate balancing mechanisms which works to maintain the right amounts of an enormous range of substances – proteins, minerals, electrolytes, as well as water – in the body. Correct balance will vary from time to time and under different circumstances such as rest, stress and disease. The processes of reabsorption are complex, moreover, not only because the cells which form the tubules must 'select' those substances which are to be reabsorbed but also because they secrete some of them back into the tubules.

The movement of both fluid and solids back and forth between the tubules and the renal blood vessels which closely surround them occurs by one of several mechanisms. Filtration into the glomerulus is caused by the hydrostatic pressure of the blood which causes water and other substances to diffuse out of the blood vessels. Some reabsorption, particularly of water, also occurs through the tubule wall by this process, although the permeability of the cells is altered by hormonal action. Thus aldosterone (see p. 82 above) and a substance called anti-diuretic hormone (ADH) secreted by the anterior pituitary gland both make the tubule more permeable to water so that the volume of urine is diminished. The mechanism by which ADH acts on tubule cells is uncertain, but aldosterone appears to increase reabsorption of sodium in the tubule, and this stimulates water reabsorption.

Water may also move by osmosis across membranous barriers such as those surrounding renal tubule cells. Osmosis occurs when a solution on one side of a semi-permeable barrier contains more dissolved molecules than does the solution on the other side. In such a situation, water (but not the dissolved molecules, because the barrier pores are too small) will move from the less dense to the more dense solution until the two are balanced. All of the solids normally dissolved in the glomerular filtrate have passed between the cells of the capillaries in the glomerulus, and can also pass through the tubule walls. Osmotic diuresis can be accomplished, however, by treatment with mannitol or urea. Both of these molecules will dissolve in plasma and will be filtered by the glomerulus, but they will not be reabsorbed through the tubules. As a result, water passes by osmosis into the tubules from the surrounding blood and tissue.

Dissolved solids also diffuse across tubule cells in both directions, depending on hydrostatic and osmotic pressure, but much of the movement of electrolytes is effected by chemical processes carried out within the cells of the tubule walls (and often in other body cells as well) which transport sodium (Na^+), potassium (K^+), hydrogen (H^+), chloride (Cl^-) and bicarbonate (HCO_3^-) from the 'outer' cell wall to the 'inner' cell wall, and across the two membranes (they are of course part of a continuous cell wall). While some of these processes involve combinations of one or more of the electrolytes with each other (e.g. $Na^+ + Cl^- \rightleftharpoons Na^+ Cl^-$, or sodium chloride; i.e. salt) in the course of the transport operation, enzymes (q.v.) such as carbonic anhydrase (see 'Acetazolamide') frequently though not always being required to effect these chemical alterations, others cannot occur without an input of energy (active transport) so that the chemical transport process is accompanied by breakdown of the energy molecules, ATP (see 'Biochemistry'). This is particularly the case with exchange transport, a special version of active transport by means of which electrolytes are 'carried' across the cellular membrane itself, a barrier which is probably no more than two molecules thick with some space between the outer and inner molecules. In exchange transport, an intracellular molecule, possibly an enzyme, plus ATP, carries Na^+, for example, from one margin of the cell wall to the other where the Na^+ is released and an atom of K^+ is picked up by the same molecule for transport on the return journey. This chemical shuttle, like other forms of active transport, can occur in all living cells.

Diuretics such as acetazolamide (q.v.) and chlorothiazide (q.v.) act by altering active-transport processes within tubule cells. Uricosurics (see 'Allopurinol') such as probenecid and sulfinpyrazone inhibit reabsorption of uric acid from the glomerular filtrate, probably by their effects on tubular transport. The anti-diuretic effects of chlorothiazide and anti-diuretic hormone may occur for similar reasons.

Electrolyte

A chemical compound which is dissociated into ions (q.v.) in solution, originally so designated because it was thought that the passage of an electric current was necessary. Subsequently it was discovered that many compounds dissociate spontaneously in solution. In medicine, the term tends to be used loosely to describe the concentration in tissue fluids of various ions; e.g., the serum 'electrolytes' – which refers to the concentration in serum (i.e. blood minus its formed elements and fibrinogen – see 'Heparin') of sodium (Na^+), potassium (K^+) and chlorine (Cl^-) ions.

Emetine

(Synthesized: R. P. Evstigneeva, *et al.*, 1950, U.S.S.R.) Emetine bismuth iodide is recommended in Great Britain, but a closely related compound, emetine hydrochloride, is preferred in the United States. Trade names: none. Administration: injection.

Classification

One of two principal constituents of ipecac, a derivative of the rhizomes of *Cephaëlis ipecacuanha* or *acuminata*, natives to Brazil and Central America. Cephaëline, the other major alkaloid derived from these plants, is much less active. Emetine is also prepared synthetically from cephaëline. The only other drug with therapeutic uses similar to those of emetine is a synthetic anti-malarial compound, chloroquine (see 'Mepacrine'), although certain drugs containing arsenic (e.g. carbarsone) or iodine (e.g. iodochlorhydroxyquin), some antibiotics (q.v.; e.g. bacitracin, erythromycin and tetracycline – q.v.), and more recent synthetics such as diloxanide furoate and metronidazole (q.v.) are useful against intestinal amoebiasis.

Therapeutic uses

Emetine and chloroquine alone are effective in the control, though not necessarily the cure, of amoebic infections outside the intestine. In addition, emetine will halt acute attacks of amoebic dysentery, which are caused by intestinal infection.

Amoebae are unicellular organisms widely distributed in fresh water and various foods. Many forms normally inhabit the human intestine, but not the one, *Entamoeba histolytica*, which causes disease. Amoebiasis occurs in every country in the world.

Like malaria and other protozoal infections, it may exist in an inactive form which reflects the vegetative cyst state of the infectious parasite. When the organism is growing and multiplying, the disease symptoms appear. Asymptomatic individuals can be carriers, and can spread the disease. To cure amoebiasis, all cysts as well as active organisms must be eliminated, but at normal dose levels emetine kills only the latter.

Entamoeba histolytica are usually taken in through the mouth, but whatever their means of ingress, they grow and become encysted not only in the intestine but in other tissues as well – especially the liver, lungs, brain and skin. Even when there is no diarrhoea, therefore, active organisms may exist in these vital organs. Thus the importance of emetine lies in the fact that, excepting for chloroquine, it is the only drug which can destroy the active, symptom-causing organisms in body tissues outside the intestines.

The compound can in fact also kill cysts, but only at dose levels dangerous to man. It causes degeneration of the nucleus and cytoplasmic elements of the amoeba, and is thought to interfere with multiplication of the active trophozoites.

Side effects
Emetine is very irritating, and must be kept away from the eyes. Indeed, its oral administration is impossible because the drug irritates the mucous lining of the gastrointestinal tract. More important, however, are the possible toxic reactions caused by the agent. Gastrointestinal effects are frequent and include nausea, vomiting and severe diarrhoea, which must of course be distinguished from the dysenteric diarrhoea caused by the infectious amoebae. Dizziness, faintness and headache may occur. Weakness, aching and tender muscles, mild sensory disturbances, tremor, oedema and pain may result from muscular irritation. The most serious toxic effects, however, occur in the heart and circulatory system. They may include a fall in blood pressure, abnormally rapid heartbeat, dilation of the heart, heart failure and death. Thus, the drug must be used with great care, especially with children and pregnant women, and with patients suffering from weaknesses of the heart or kidneys. For patients with heart trouble, chloroquine is normally used before emetine.

The drug remains in the body from six to eight weeks so that there is a danger of cumulative effects. However, most untoward reactions commonly experienced are mild; even if emetine therapy continues, they may disappear, suggesting that the body develops a tolerance for the compound.

In an effort both to broaden the amoebicidal effectiveness of the drug, and to reduce the dangers arising from its toxicity, emetine may be given with chloroquine, and with oxytetracycline (see 'Tetracycline') when treatment is directed against intestinal amoebiasis.

Enzyme

A protein catalyst formed by living cells.* The word derives from a Greek expression meaning 'leaven', and reflects the early recognition that yeast catalyses the fermentation of sugars to ethyl alcohol (q.v.) and carbon dioxide. In fact, this organic process requires the participation of several yeast enzymes. Similarly, however, it has long been recognized that gastric and pancreatic juices catalyse the digestion of proteins in food. The original products engaged in these chemical reactions, sugars and proteins in the examples given, are called substrates.

Proteins (see 'Biochemistry') are molecules composed of long chains of some twenty amino acids in varying combinations, linked by peptide bonds. Literally millions of different proteins exist in nature, and the vast majority of those which are known are enzymes. The numbers of enzymes synthesized by human body cells have not yet been counted.

These protein catalysts perform functions similar to those of any chemical catalyst; that is, they cause possible chemical recombinations to occur which would either take place much more slowly without them, or not at all, and they are not themselves chemically altered at the end of the process. But biological catalysts (enzymes) possess three qualities to a much higher degree than do their non-biological analogues: activity, specificity and efficiency.

Sucrose (glucose and fructose combined in one molecule) and other disaccharides can be split in water (hydrolysed) in the presence of a mineral acid such as hydrochloric acid, if the acid concentration and temperature are high. The enzyme invertase

* Adapted from George H. Bell, J. N. Davidson and H. Scarborough, *Textbook of Physiology and Biochemistry*, Edinburgh and London, 1968, p. 109.

accomplishes the same thing at room temperature (i.e. without the extra energy supplied by heat) with $\frac{1}{100,000}$ the amount of catalyst.

Non-biological catalysts tend to lack specificity. Thus, acids assist the hydrolysis not only of disaccharides but also of polysaccharides, proteins and certain fats; they catalyse many other reactions as well. Two of the pancreatic enzymes, trypsin and chymotrypsin, catalyse the breakdown of food proteins, but trypsin breaks only the bond between the carboxyl group (CO) which links lysine or arginine to another amino acid, while chymotrypsin attacks the bond between the carboxyl group of an aromatic amino acid (one containing a benzene ring) and any other amino acid (though this section is inhibited if another carboxyl group is physically near by). Thus:

(Bell, Davidson and Scarborough, *op. cit.*, p. 111.)

This remarkable enzymic specificity applies not only to the substrate but also to the reactions catalysed. Many substrates are metabolized into more than one substance by normal cells. Each of these reactions requires the intervention of a different enzyme even though the substrate, the original reaction product, is the same.

Both because they are so specific and because of their high activity, enzymes are almost a hundred per cent efficient. There is practically no wastage of substrates, however many steps the biosynthetic process entails.

All of these qualities stem from the physico–chemical characteristics of enzyme molecules. Although a protein is in the first instance a long chain of amino acids (probably no fewer than twenty and as many as five hundred) connected by peptide bonds, the molecule possesses at least one other essential characteristic, probably two and possibly three. These are called structures.

The primary structure of a protein is the amino–acid chain itself:

$$
\begin{array}{ccc}
O & R & H \\
\| & | & | \\
C & CH & N \\
| \diagdown \diagup | & | \diagup \\
\diagup N \diagdown & C & CH \\
| & \| & | \\
H & O & R
\end{array}
$$

R = an amino acid

Secondary structure occurs in most but not all known proteins. It is the helical conformation taken up by the molecule as a result of hydrogen bonds (i.e. a loosely formed link between a hydrogen atom and an oxygen atom mediated by the single hydrogen electron) established between amino acids with the necessary free H and O atoms at regular intervals along the chain.

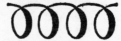

The heavier line is above and the lighter line is beneath the plane of the page

This helical formation may also be recognized as the basic structure of the genetic molecule, DNA, which is not a protein, however.

Regardless of whether the protein folds into a helix, it will display a tertiary structure. Atoms in one amino acid will attract or repel atoms in other amino acids along the chain, and will form loose links such as hydrogen bonds between some of those between which attraction occurs, according to fundamental chemical laws. The chain will, therefore, twist and fold about itself like a rubber band rubbed between two hands. Obviously, the resultant shapes will vary enormously; in fact, each protein takes up a unique conformation, governed in the main by its primary structure.

This tertiary structure, containing two helices, is imaginary. It serves to illustrate the reason for the specificity of an enzyme, however. The deep cleft in the top right of the molecule provides a series of points at which a longish molecule of specific (imaginary) substrate could become attached to the enzyme by various loose links such as hydrogen bonds. Held in this fashion, the 'head' of the substrate molecule is brought into contact with the active site (dotted circle) consisting of one or more amino acids (here at least two) on the strand(s) within the active site.

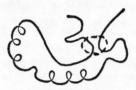

There a chemical reaction occurs; for example, one or more atoms on the 'head' of the substrate molecule are detached from the substrate because they are (temporarily) more strongly attracted to the enzymal amino acids. Detachment of the atom or atoms alters the chemical characteristics of the substrate so that its bonds with the enzyme break and, thus changed, it is released. The disappearance of the rest of the molecule simultaneously alters the characteristics of the atoms which have remained attached to the active site, and they too are now released, thus returning the enzyme to its pre-reaction condition.

The imaginary enzyme has thus split a substrate molecule. It must be realized that under normal circumstances the reaction described above takes place so rapidly that it would be almost impossible to see it even if the atoms involved were not far below the resolving power of the most powerful microscopes available. Descriptions of actual molecular events catalysed by enzymes are deduced from knowledge of the pre- and post-reaction products and of the laws of chemistry.

In addition to splitting substrate molecules, enzymes combine atoms and molecules, transfer atoms from one molecule to another, transfer electrons between atoms, rearrange the component atoms of a molecule, and link two molecules at the expense of the breakdown of a third. All of these reactions require that the substrate 'fit' the enzyme in such a way that the appropriate substrate atoms are juxtaposed to the enzymal active site. Any alteration in the tertiary structure of an enzyme due to heat, chemicals such as drugs or some disease states will cause the catalysed reaction to stop (cf. the analogous linkage between acetylcholine and its receptor site, under 'Atropine').

Some proteins also display quaternary structure, a conformation in which the functional molecule consists of two or four identical or very similar proteins whose tertiary structures are such as to form bonds between themselves. Insulin (q.v.), which is a protein but not an enzyme, consists of two chains tightly linked together by disulphide (double sulphur–hydrogen) bonds. Haemoglobin, the principal constituent of red blood cells – also a protein though not an enzyme – has four chains, two of one structure and two of another, each of which contains a haem group, a small molecule the central atom of which is an iron ion (q.v.; an iron atom lacking either two or three electrons, and therefore double- or triple-positively charged). The haem molecule within each of the four linked proteins takes up atmospheric oxygen (O_2), and releases it to the tissues in exchange for carbon dioxide. It is known as a prosthetic group, a non-protein molecule which is an integral part of the larger molecule without which the larger molecule could not function. Enzymes may also contain prosthetic groups, some of which are formed from vitamins (q.v.) such as thiamine.

Enzymes with quaternary structure may be isoenzymes, a term which means that the enzyme exists normally in two or more forms which have the same catalytic activity although they are chemically different. This usually occurs because, like haemoglobin, the isoenzymes consist of four units of two different protein types (A and B) which may form different combinations within the whole enzyme molecule: AAAA, AAAB, AABB, ABBB, BBBB.

Prosthetic groups are actually parts of enzymal molecules. Coenzymes, on the other hand, may best be thought of as small, non-protein molecules which are separate from the enzyme molecule, but without which the enzyme cannot perform its catalytic role. For example, adenosine triphosphate (ATP), the energy-storage molecule (see 'Biochemistry'), is also a co-enzyme in a great many reactions which require free energy, or themselves create energy. This energy is released by the breaking of a phosphate bond, so that ATP becomes adenosine diphosphate (ADP), or energy is stored by formation of ATP from ADP. In each such reaction, the phosphate group is transferred from ATP to the substrate, or from the substrate to ADP. Other coenzymes such as nicotinamide-adenine dinucleotide (NAD) and flavin-adenine dinucleotide (FAD), are biosynthesized from vitamins (q.v.), in these cases, nicotinic acid and riboflavine, respectively – both B-type vitamins.

Very few cellular chemical reactions occur without the intercession of an enzyme. Since the symptoms of disease are the result of chemical disturbances in the body (this is demonstrably true of at least some 'mental' diseases, too), malfunctioning enzymes may be the root cause of the illness. Even when this cannot be proven, as in the vast majority of diseases at present, it must be admitted, it is nevertheless the case that manipulation of enzymes can sometimes eliminate the symptoms. Thus, carbonic anhydrase inhibitors are useful against gout (see 'Allopurinol') and hypertension (see 'Chlorothiazide'). Monoamine oxidase inhibitors are anti-depressants, and serve other useful therapeutic purposes. Adrenaline (q.v.) exerts its 'natural' as against its pharmacological effects by stimulating formation of an enzyme, phosphorylase, which catalyses the breakdown of glycogen into glucose. The sulphonamides (q.v.), furthermore, selectively inhibit the growth of some bacteria which must synthesize an essential coenzyme, folic acid, while mammalian cells can utilize only pre-formed folic acid (as a vitamin) from food. Penicillin (q.v.) and other antibiotics (q.v.) inhibit enzymes essential to the formation of bacterial cell walls. An understanding of enzymes and enzyme chemistry is clearly essential to modern pharmacology.

Ephedrine

Trade names: over thirty-five in Great Britain alone. Administration: oral; topical, in creams, eye-drops, nasal sprays and inhalers; by injection for treatment of acute fall in blood pressure.

Classification
Derived from *Ephedra equisetina* and some other plants, the compound had been in use in Chinese medicine for centuries before it was introduced into modern western pharmacopoeias

(1924). A synthetic product, racephedrine hydrochloride, is also available.

Like adrenaline (q.v.) and amphetamine (q.v.), ephedrine is a sympathomimetic drug; that is, its actions mimic some of the effects naturally arising from stimulation of the sympathetic division of the autonomic or involuntary nervous system (see 'Adrenaline').

The similarities between the actions of ephedrine and adrenaline are so great that it is worth while to call attention to their differences: ephedrine can be administered orally, it acts for a longer period (seven to ten times as long), it has more pronounced effects on the central nervous system (CNS; amphetamine has stronger CNS effects than either ephedrine or adrenaline), but it is otherwise less powerful.

Therapeutic uses

Ephedrine is useful for treatment of acute asthmatic attacks and for chronic asthma. Its prolonged activity also makes it suitable for the control of hay fever and similar allergic disorders, and as a nasal decongestant.

The compound is employed to treat a heart condition called the Stokes-Adams syndrome, a severe heart block which causes fainting and possibly death. Ephedrine may also be used to prevent subsequent attacks. The drug may be employed to raise blood pressure, particularly during spinal anaesthesia, but not during general anaesthesia, because the anaesthetic substances tend to make the heart more sensitive to erratic rhythms which can be induced by ephedrine.

Because of its stimulatory effect on the brain, the agent is useful in a condition called narcolepsy where the patient falls asleep involuntarily and without warning. It is also employed to relax the pupils of the eye, to treat urinary incontinence and enuresis and to relax the uterus in order to reduce the pain of menstruation.

Side effects

These are similar to those of adrenaline, though less severe. The CNS effects can produce insomnia and irritability. To combat these conditions, a barbiturate (see 'Phenobarbitone') is usually administered simultaneously if ephedrine is to be used over a period of time.

The compound is a non-catechol amine, lacking the hydroxyl (OH) groups which occur on the benzene ring (see 'Biochemistry') in adrenaline:

$$\langle\bigcirc\rangle\!-\!\underset{OH}{CH}\!-\!\underset{CH_3}{CH}\!-\!\underset{CH_3}{NH}$$

Its activity no doubt arises in the main from its chemical similarity to noradrenaline, the chemical substance which transmits nerve impulses between nerve ends or between nerve ends and muscle cells in the sympathetic nervous system. Thus, ephedrine is known as a spasmolytic agent, and is used as a bronchodilator, because it acts on sympathetic alpha-receptors to relax smooth muscle such as that found in the bronchial tubes. Its usefulness against Stokes-Adams disease, on the other hand, derives from its activity on sympathetic beta-receptors in the heart. This heart action is thought to be the major cause of the increased blood pressure mediated by the drug, although this effect may also be due to action of the agent on the smooth muscles which constrict peripheral blood vessels. In any event, because the constriction of nasal blood vessels tends to open the air passages in the nose, it is principally this action which gives ephedrine its familiar usefulness as a nasal decongestant. Part of the effect on peripheral blood vessels may also derive from the ability of the drug to cause the release of noradrenaline from neurons; it would then be the natural transmitter which causes the muscular constriction of the peripheral blood vessels rather than any direct drug action, although both mechanisms could be in operation at the same time. Because of the complexity of its actions on various tissues, the behaviour of the drug remains to be clarified.

Ethyl alcohol (ethanol)

Although ethyl alcohol in the form of wine and beer has apparently been used since history began, distilling was introduced to Europe by the Arabs. Alchemists looked upon the new beverages as the elixir of life, whence came the word 'whisky' (Gaelic: *usquebaugh*, 'water of life').

Therapeutic uses

According to one leading textbook of pharmacology, 'the therapeutic value of alcohol is much more limited than is its social value'.* Nevertheless, it has its uses as a drug, too. As a

*Louis S. Goodman and A. Gilman, *op. cit.*, p. 143.

solvent, it can wash away the oil which causes oak and ivy poisoning, provided it is used early and thoroughly. It cools the skin as it evaporates, and affords a pleasant and effective sponge bath during fever. Its slight irritant effect on skin explains its inclusion in liniments, and it can reduce the incidence of bed sores. It is a cheap and potent bactericidal skin disinfectant, but should not be used to disinfect open wounds because it dehydrates and injures cells, and because it can cause the formation of a blood serum clot which tends to protect bacteria.

Alcohol effectively relieves extreme and persistent pain from angina pectoris, certain forms of neuralgia and inoperable cancers, and tuberculous laryngitis. For these purposes, it must be injected locally. It can be useful, also, for controlling acute oedema or fluid collection in the lungs resulting from heart failure. For this purpose, it must be inhaled as a gas.

In convalescent and elderly patients, the compound can improve both appetite and digestion, and it can reduce colic and flatulence. As a treatment for the common cold, it has only one purpose: to make the patient sleepy enough so that he will stay in bed. Similarly, it can be an anti-insomniac in convalescent patients. That alcohol is a general anaesthetic, common experience suggests; it is not used for this purpose under normal surgical circumstances for two major reasons: it is very slowly eliminated from the body by comparison with the usual anaesthetics (see 'Halothane'), and the dose required for anaesthesia is very close to that which can cause dangerous respiratory malfunction. Lesser amounts can of course cause euphoria which changes the patient's reaction to pain in much the same way as does morphine.

There is growing evidence that alcohol intoxication can favourably influence certain types of learning. It seems probable that to remember something learned under the influence of alcohol, a similar state of inebriation is most effective. *In vino veritas* contains more than a little truth.

Side effects
The most prominent of these can scarcely be called undesirable, yet drunkenness is not a therapeutically useful effect in and of itself. It is of course a result of the effects of alcohol on the central nervous system (CNS), and it is these effects ('Chemistry and physiology', below) which probably explain the addictive-

ness of the drug, though not the development of tolerance to it in the sense that more and more of it appears to be required to achieve the same results. Addictiveness is demonstrated by the withdrawal symptoms coincident upon abstention; these may range from 'hangover' to insomnia, the 'shakes', the 'jitters' and delirium tremens. As a drug of abuse, alcohol is far and away the most significant problem in western society, both from the physiological and from the social standpoints. However, there is no evidence that alcoholism is an inherited characteristic (though mental factors predisposing to it may be) or that miscarriages among alcoholic women are more frequent than among non-alcoholics (though, again, alcoholics do have more children, thus increasing the likelihood of miscarriage).

Many of the effects such as neuritis, ophthalmic malfunctions, gastrointestinal problems and cirrhosis of the liver previously ascribed to alcohol poisoning are now thought to occur because of the malnutrition and vitamin deficiencies which can accompany alcoholism. But excessive doses of the drug can indeed cause death due to pneumonia and to increased cranial pressure. Alcohol should certainly not be used by people with ulcers, hyperacidity or epilepsy, and probably not by those with liver or kidney disease. (For a brief discussion of methyl alcohol, see the end of this entry.)

Chemistry and physiology

Ethyl alcohol (C_2H_5OH) is absorbed from the stomach and more rapidly from the small intestine. It is widely and fairly evenly distributed throughout all tissues and fluids, and ninety-eight per cent is completely oxidized (see 'Biochemistry') within the body. The rate of oxidation (which means the rate at which the drug is broken down so that its effects cease) is related to time and not to dose, although starvation lowers the rate, while insulin (q.v.) increases it, and there is preliminary evidence that fructose (fruit sugar) in high enough doses can also produce an increase. Food reduces the rate of absorption from the stomach, though probably not from the small intestine; it does not appear to affect the rate of oxidation.

Oxidation occurs chiefly in the liver where an enzyme (q.v.), alcohol dehydrogenase, begins the process by converting alcohol to acetaldehyde (see 'Disulfiram'). This compound is in turn converted either directly or via the intermediate form of acetic acid (fruit sugar) to a substance called acetyl coenzyme A (see 'Vitamin'), an essential metabolite in the intracellular breakdown of carbohydrates. However, the breakdown of carbohydrates by the liver is decreased in the presence of alcohol, and there is some increase in the production of metabolites such as fatty acids which are normally further broken down by liver cells. It is thought that these events occur because the enzyme, alcohol dehydrogenase, utilizes nicotinamide adenine dinucleotide (NAD) as an 'acceptor' molecule for the hydrogen atoms removed from the hydroxyl (OH) group in the initial oxidation of alcohol, thus decreasing the amount of NAD available for the other metabolic processes normally carried out in liver cells. This may be part of the biochemistry behind the fat deposits in the livers of chronic alcoholics which appear to lead to cirrhosis (see below).

Nevertheless, the breakdown of alcohol does provide immediate energy, just as does the more usual catabolism of carbohydrates. Thus, the alcoholic requires less food, and eats less. The effect of alcohol in large amounts on the stomach lining is very irritating, which probably explains the relatively high incidence of stomach ulcers in chronic alcoholics who do not mix food with their drink. Similarly, the constipation suffered by alcoholics is caused by the absence of food mass. Conversely, diarrhoea may be caused by a lack of vitamins (q.v.), and this deficiency can contribute to many more serious disturbances such as cirrhosis of the liver. The familiar warmth which accompanies a drink probably occurs because of enhanced blood flow in the skin and gut, a central and possibly an endocrine-stimulating (see discussion under 'Hormone') effect of alcohol, rather than because of the caloric energy output.

Alcohol is a depressant; any stimulatory effect it appears to have occurs because it first depresses a primitive central co-ordinating mechanism in the brain, the reticular activating system, thus freeing the cortex and other higher (as opposed to primitive) centres from regulation. The euphoria, as well as the disturbances in mental and motor processes, arise from this suppression of brain co-ordination. If mental inhibition does prevent a person from carrying out a task, alcohol may 'unblock' him, but on the whole, it is believed that, with the possible exception noted above in connexion with learning ('Therapeutic uses'), alcohol does not improve mental ability. The more alcohol there is in the blood, the greater will be the disturbance of CNS functions; i.e. the drunker the imbiber. Yet, curiously, the symptoms of drunkenness are more apparent when the blood level is rising towards a peak than when it is falling away from it.

The molecular mechanisms of action of alcohol in the CNS are unclear. Evidence has been presented that in the body some acetaldehyde may react with adrenaline (q.v.) so that the acetaldehyde is converted into very small amounts of a substance called tetrahydroisoquinoline. This compound is found in the hallucinogen, mescal, derived from the peyote cactus. The implication is that the CNS effects of alcohol may occur because a small amount of it is utilized by the body to biosynthesize a hallucinogen.

Methyl alcohol (methanol, meths, red biddy, wood alcohol; CH_3OH) is a frank poison. It is oxidized to formaldehyde, which probably causes the blindness so frequent after the ingestion of the compound, and formic acid. The latter quickly and severely disrupts the acid-base balance of the body by acidifying the blood, and can rapidly kill. The first order of treatment is rectification of the acidosis by dosage with alkali such as sodium bicarbonate. Ethyl alcohol itself can be a useful antidote: the oxidative mechanism for ethanol and methanol are the same, but the former competes more successfully for the enzyme, alcohol dehydrogenase, and prevents formation of formaldehyde and formic acid from the latter. This also explains why meths drinkers who take some wine, beer, spirits or even rubbing alcohol (seventy per cent ethanol) may be partially protected against themselves.

5-Fluorouracil

(Heidelberger, *et al.*, 1957, U.S.) Trade name: none; the drug is not available for general prescription. Administration: intravenous injection.

Classification
The first of a series of synthetic anti-tumour agents developed from rational biochemical predictions as to its probable mechanism of action ('Chemistry and Physiology', below). The compound is closely related chemically to an essential constituent of intracellular molecules (deoxyribonucleic acid, DNA) which carry genetic information from one cell generation to the next. Its usefulness has given rise to several similar compounds which are employed clinically: 5-iododeoxyuridine and 6-azauridine (a related compound which is also used for the treatment of psoriasis; see 'Fluocinolone acetonide'), 5-fluoromethyldeoxyuridine and cytosine arabinoside. 5-Fluorouracil is closely related chemically to 5-fluorodeoxyuridine, which may be a less toxic drug under some circumstances.

Therapeutic uses
The agent may slow the growth of cancers of the breast and gastrointestinal tract, and is considered to be moderately useful in the treatment of cancer of the ovary, cervix, urinary bladder and of the throat and middle ear. It is not a cancer cure. Reports

indicate that up to thirty per cent of patients who have received the drug have been benefited by it. In the most successful treatments, temporary relief up to five years has been achieved, and in breast cancer, survival time has been increased by as much as one year. While such results are relatively limited achievements, they warrant continued use of a dangerously toxic drug, as well as hope for improvement in the treatment of this melancholy disease.

One of the limitations on the use of the drug is the tendency of tumour cells to develop resistance to its action. The reason for this is unclear, though it seems that some of the tumour cells are either impermeable to the agent, or incapable of metabolizing (see 'Metabolism') it into the chemical form it must take in order to kill the cell. These resistant cells then multiply so that cancer growth continues.

Side effects

The cell-destroying action of the compound can also affect normal bone marrow, lymphoid tissue (the system of tubes and glands which conduct body fluids to the bloodstream and also engage in primary immune-defence reactions such as the production of antibodies), mucous membranes, hair- and nail-producing cells and other body cells which proliferate rapidly. Toxic effects usually appear first as loss of appetite and nausea, inflammation in the mouth and diarrhoea. Other oral and gastrointestinal disturbances follow, and are succeeded by blood disturbances, loss of hair and skin and nervous disorders. 5-Fluorouracil and 5-fluorodeoxyuridine are believed to have been responsible for the deaths of about three per cent of patients who have received them.

Chemistry and physiology

Like actinomycin D (q.v.), azathioprine (q.v.), chlorambucil (q.v.) and methotrexate (q.v.), 5-fluorouracil disrupts normal cellular metabolism. It interferes with biosynthesis of the nucleic acids, deoxyribonucleic acid (DNA) and, to a lesser extent, ribonucleic acid (RNA), without which the cell can neither transmit genetic characteristics to the next generation (DNA), nor grow and function properly (RNA). Thus, the compound kills the more rapidly proliferating cells, and its usefulness derives from the fact that some cancer cells grow and divide more quickly than most normal body cells.

Both DNA and RNA are composed of two sorts of bases, pyrimidines and purines, plus a pentose sugar (ribose; see 'Biochemistry') and a phosphate. The pyrimidine bases (there are essentially only two in each nucleic acid: cytosine and thymine in DNA and cytosine and uracil in RNA, just as there are only two purines in each) have the general structure:

$$3N \underset{2}{\overset{4}{\diamond}} \begin{matrix} 5 \\ N \, 6 \end{matrix}$$

The numbers identify specific C and N atomic positions. Thus, the 5 in the name of the compound indicates that the fluorine atom appears in the fifth position, as shown:

$$\text{HN} \diamond \text{F (5-fluorouracil structure)}$$

In the biosynthesis of the pyrimidines required for formation of nucleic acids, 5-fluorouracil (after being converted metabolically to a ribonucleotide; i.e. the base, pentose and phosphate, and subsequently, a deoxynucleotide) is believed to inhibit an enzyme (q.v.), thymidilate synthetase, which catalyses an essential step in the synthesis of thymine. It would, therefore, be an anti-metabolite of one of the constituent bases of DNA. Since thymine is unique in DNA (being replaced by uracil in RNA), the search for an effective pyrimidine analogue as an anti-metabolite concentrated on precisely this pathway. It is also probable, however, that the agent replaces uracil in newly formed RNA, thus damaging that vital cell constituent as well.

Fluocinolone acetonide

(Synthesized: Mills, Bowers, Djerassi, Ringold and Zderic, 1958, U.S.) Trade name: Synalar; with antibiotics: Synalar-N, Synalar-C; also Synandone. Administration: External application as creams, ointments, gels or solution.

Classification
A synthetic anti-inflammatory compound related to corticosteroids (see 'Hydrocortisone') but with special chemical modification to enhance activity when applied externally. In terms of equivalent concentrations fluocinolone acetonide is probably the

most active of the preparations available. Related compounds include triamcinolone acetonide, betamethasone, flurandrenolone, flumethasone pivalate, beclomethasone dipropionate and flucortolone, as well as hydrocortisone (q.v.) and prednisolone.

Therapeutic uses
In different forms of skin disease, the clinical picture varies from the angry red wet acute condition with breakage of the skin surface on the one hand (figuratively speaking) to the silvery scaling dry patches of psoriasis on the other. Parenthetically it might be noted that there is a large nervous element in psoriasis, and several of the 'miracle' cures of what was thought to be leprosy in the Bible might well be explained by a semi-hypnotic elimination of the nervous element. The topical corticosteroid preparations, that is, those used externally, are advocated for most of these diseases, and many authors have stated that their introduction, and in particular the availability of the newer steroids containing the chemical fluorine in the molecule, have revolutionized the treatment of these disorders. While there can be no doubt about their efficacy in acute disorders, opinion is divided regarding their use where the skin disease is long-standing (chronic). The disease can reappear after the time required has passed for the steroid to be completely eliminated from the skin in which some of the available compounds persist for a remarkably long period; for example, fluocinolone acetonide can be demonstrated in skin up to at least sixteen days after its last application. None the less, even in these cases the use of the compounds is justified, if only to produce a quick improvement of acute episodes to allow further treatment with more conventional measures.

Combination products of steroid with antibiotic (q.v.) or antiseptic are also available, and are frequently used where infection is thought to be a part of the clinical picture. There is less justification for such blunderbuss therapy, if only because of the incidence of sensitization which is seen with neomycin, one of the most commonly used antibiotics.

Topical steroids can be used successfully in keloid, where there is overgrowth of hard scar tissue following a skin wound, changes which can be reversed or diminished by localized injection of the steroid into the actual scar. In these conditions the steroids are presumably acting by decreasing the activity of the tissue fibroblasts, special cells which form the fibres of the connective tissue immediately below the skin, and which also form the scar tissue of wounds. Topical steroids are for application to the exterior of the body. However, what is not always realized is that the exterior extends from the mouth and nose through the body to the anus also, and it is not surprising therefore that certain 'topical' preparations are available for the treatment of such areas. These are particularly for ulceration in the mouth, and for alleviation of allergic rhinitis (hay fever). These drugs are thought to be useful in the treatment of hay fever because their action is similar to that of systemic steroids; they suppress the cellular reaction to an antigen–antibody reaction (see 'Azathioprine'), the antigen in this case being pollen, or a similar irritant.

Side effects

With proper usage these are minimal or absent. However, application over wide areas of the body, particularly if carried out under polythene wrapping to increase absorption (occlusion), may lead to local changes in the form of thinning of the skin or to general changes due to absorption of significant amounts of steroid, for example, mild decrease in function of the adrenal glands. Rarely, use of these compounds in psoriasis may lead to the formation of new areas of involved skin.

Chemistry and physiology

Most of the modern topical steroids have a fluorine substitution on the basic chemical structure, generally in the 9α-position (see 'Hormones') which is known to enhance the anti-inflammatory activity of corticosteroids (see 'Hydrocortisone'). In addition many have a special substitution – a 16,17-acetonide group, which is known to enhance penetration across the skin barrier.

acetonide

Such enhancement of penetration has been shown with the use of radioactive compounds, and also by means of a specialized test carried out on human volunteers. The molecular mechanism of action of these drugs is not clear, but it is believed that they counteract the effect of histamine and prostaglandin (q.v.) release by cells in the skin. Histamine release would explain the classical features of inflammation seen in acute skin disease: *Calor* (heat), *rubor* (redness) and *tumor* (swelling), the last mentioned being caused by dilation of blood vessels which makes them leak fluid into tissues, and stimulation of local nerve endings resulting in the fourth classical symptom of inflammation, *dolor* (pain and itching). Certainly, such changes can be produced experimentally in normal skin and in tissue culture by suitable irritation. At the cellular level, these changes can be shown to be accompanied by increased permeability of an intracellular organelle called a lysosome which contains breakdown enzymes, normally employed in the removal of unwanted molecules from the cell. Increased lysosomal permeability releases the enzymes contained in them. Similarly, mitochondria, the energy-producing organelles of the cells, may become more permeable. The result of these structural changes could be a disruption in cellular metabolism (q.v.). By maintaining the cells structurally and chemically intact, some of the newer topical steroids can reverse these changes, and this could explain their effectiveness in treatment of acute skin diseases. However, their mechanism of action in chronic skin diseases – diseases such as psoriasis – is not understood.

Guanethidine

(Muell, Maxwell and Plummer, 1957, U.S.) Trade name: Ismelin. Administration: oral in tablets, and less often by injection.

Classification
Representative of a group of drugs that achieve their effects by depressing the function of a part of the sympathetic nervous system (see 'Adrenaline', and 'Chemistry and physiology', below). Bretylium is the only clinically useful drug with some chemical similarities, however.

Therapeutic uses
Guanethidine is used principally to combat the symptoms of severe high blood pressure (hypertension), though it no more cures this poorly understood condition than does any other known treatment. It acts too slowly to be useful against sudden acute rises in blood pressure, and it is frequently given with one of the thiazides (see 'Chlorothiazide') in order to reduce the dosage required.

The agent has also been used to control a form of sudden

erratic speeding up of heartbeat. It is less frequently administered to patients with overactive thyroid, presumably to reduce their blood pressure, and to control certain skin diseases.

Side effects

The most common effect of the drug is a severe fall in blood pressure when the patient stands erect (postural hypotension), especially after sleep or exercise, in hot weather or with consumption of alcohol. This condition can be dangerous, and because the drug works slowly and remains in the body for a relatively long period, precautions against postural hypotension are essential.

Diarrhoea is also a common though less serious and more easily controlled side effect. Others may include dizziness and weakness, shallow breathing, fainting, rapid heartbeat and oedema (accumulation of excess body fluid in tissues). There have been rare reports of kidney infection, which is possible if kidney function is poor to begin with, and nausea, vomiting, vision disturbances, depression, increased frequency of urination and failure of ejaculation (though not impotence *per se*).

Chemistry and physiology

Both the side effects and the therapeutic uses of guanethidine derive from its effects on certain nerves. Between the central nervous system (CNS) – the brain and spinal cord – and peripheral organs, substations called ganglia provide cross-over linkages between parts of the autonomic nervous system. Nerves from the spinal cord enter a ganglion from which additional nerves carry the message further to the specialized receptor cells of muscle in the heart and stomach or of the hormone-synthesizing tissue in the adrenals, as well as other organs. It is this latter group of nerves, the post-ganglionic fibres, which guanethidine depresses.

These sympathetic nerves transmit their impulses to the effector cells by means of a chemical called noradrenaline (see 'Adrenaline') which they synthesize, store and release under appropriate stimulation. Guanethidine may act in part because it dissipates the stores of noradrenaline from the post-ganglionic adrenergic fibres. This could explain the fact that before the drug exerts its anti-hypertensive action, it may cause a transient rise in blood pressure; that is, the muscle cells in arterioles responsible for maintenance of peripheral circulatory pressure are excessively stimulated by the sudden release of noradrenaline. The action of the drug to depress or block nervous regulation of blood pressure probably explains the postural hypotension that may accompany its use ('Side effects', above).

Guanethidine does not appear to compete with noradrenaline for the molecular receptors in the effector cells. Both types of adrenergic receptors appear to be first stimulated and then depressed by the drug. Then presumably because of the relative disappearance of noradrenaline from the post-ganglionic fibres, and the resultant absence of the transmitter from the system, the receptor sites become supersensitive to noradrenaline, and to compounds related to it such as amphetamine (q.v.) and adrenaline (q.v.).

Just how these effects are induced by the drug, or what combination of them produces both its desirable and its undesirable actions is not clear. All three effects – release of noradrenaline, the resultant sympathetic nervous activity and the eventual supersensitivity of effector cells – occur in varying combinations under different circumstances in individual patients.

Hallucinogen (Psychedelic, Psychotomimetic, Psychotogen)

One of a class of drugs that produce hallucinations, though this is neither the only effect of these compounds nor in all cases their most significant effect. Depending on dose and the condition of the patient, the drugs can cause anxiety, delusions, paranoia, depersonalization and other symptoms common to certain psychotic states, particularly schizophrenia. The hallucinations, however, are almost always visual, whereas schizophrenic hallucinations may be aural.

It was the striking similarities between the effects of these agents and the symptoms of mental disease that aroused scientific interest in the hallucinogens after the Second World War. The drugs, especially lysergic acid diethylamide (LSD), seemed to hold out two hopes in an otherwise dreary therapeutic landscape: by using them in animals, it might be possible to develop models for the study of mental abnormalities in humans, and by noting their effects on natural substances in test-tubes and in animal models, it might be possible to identify biochemical disturbances that are associated with mental disease. Unfortunately, neither procedure has been fruitful.

The hallucinogens are not a clearcut group of drugs either in terms of their chemistry or of their pharmacological effects. Substances as diverse as mepacrine (q.v.), cocaine (q.v.), corticosteroids (see 'Hormones'), nitrous oxide and ethyl ether (see 'Halothane'), sunflower seeds and nutmeg in the right doses and conditions can produce illusions and hallucinations. All hallucinogens appear to act in the brain, however. As a class, they all induce altered perceptual states that are otherwise experienced only in dreams or during religious excitement. Three types of chemical compounds are customarily called hallucinogens: amphetamine (q.v.)-like drugs, exemplified by mescaline; indole-amines, especially LSD; and cannabis.

Mescaline is the principal active ingredient of the peyote cactus. The plant has been eaten as a religious ceremony by American and Mexican Indians in much the same symbolic manner as the wafer and wine are used in the Christian com-munion – though with somewhat different subjective effects. Mescaline can produce mild symptoms such as muscle tremors as well as vivid hallucinations. It is not addictive, and does not appear to cause withdrawal symptoms.

There is some evidence (*Nature* 237:454–5, 1972) that amphetamine psychosis is caused by the metabolic (see 'Meta-bolism') alteration of amphetamine to mescaline or to a mesca-line-like substance in the liver. Amphetamine psychosis produces symptoms, including hallucinations, which are more similar to schizophrenic symptoms than those produced by LSD. The mescaline molecule differs from the amphetamine molecule by the addition to the former of three methyl (CH_3) groups. 'STP' and several other hallucinogenic compounds can be synthesized by adding methyl groups to the amphetamine molecule.

Molecules to which methyl groups have been added are said to have been methylated. Although they are in all other respects unlike amphetamine and mescaline, the second chemical type of hallucinogens are methylated versions of important biological molecules, the indoleamines. Even LSD, which was synthesized in 1939, contains within its molecule a portion similar to the putative transmitter of nervous impulses between some nerve cells in the brain, 5-hydroxytryptamine (5-HT, serotonin; see 'Phenelzine'), which is an indoleamine. Psilocybin and psilocin, the active ingredients of the Mexican 'magic mushroom', and other compounds such as dimethyl tryptamine (DMT) are structurally similar molecules. Unlike other hallucinogens, DMT is inactive by mouth. LSD is about 100 times more potent than psilocybin and psilocin, and 4,000 times more potent than mescaline. Afficionados claim, however, that the 'trip' sustained on the natural products is pleasanter and less likely to be painful than the 'acid trip'.

The mechanism of action of these compounds is not clear. It was originally thought that the indoleamines such as LSD must somehow impair the natural function of 5-HT. In rats, LSD slightly increases brain levels of 5-HT. Other compounds which are known to reduce the amount of 5-HT in the brain enhance the effects of LSD. Monoamine oxidase inhibitors (see 'Phenelzine') increase 5-HT levels and diminish the effects of LSD. But the amphetamine-like hallucinogens such as mescaline bear no resemblance to 5-HT. They are chemically related, however, to another putative transmitter of nervous impulses between some brain nerve cells, noradrenaline (see 'Adrenaline'), and both the indoleamines and the amphetamine-like agents alter stores of noradrenaline in the brain. There are enzymes (q.v.) common to the biosynthesis of both 5-HT and noradrenaline, furthermore, so that the two chemical types of hallucinogen could in theory work at an enzymatic crossroad that would affect the quantities of both 5-HT and noradrenaline. It is now believed that these hallucinogens work at the same brain cells because their structural similarities are more important than their chemical differences. In any event, the amount of the chemicals being changed by the drugs may be very small, a few molecules more or less in a few nerve cells. There is even evidence that the neurons on which the drugs act are located in the hypothalamus (see 'Hormone') and have direct connexions to the visual as well as the emotional centres of the brain. (These centres are discussed briefly in connection with the tri-cyclic anti-depressant drugs; see 'Imipramine'.)

Like mescaline, LSD has been used for the study of schizophrenia and in the psychotherapy of neurotic patients. LSD has also been used to treat chronic alcoholism. Perhaps its most bizarre and humane value, however, is to still the fear and anxiety and diminish the pain of patients suffering terminal cancer and other fatal conditions.

The effects of LSD appear within a few minutes. They may include a period of tension followed by relaxation, perceptual changes and slowing of time. Some users experience nausea, fever and an urge to urinate. Marked hallucinations begin in an hour or two and may last four to five hours. They may include synaesthesia, the crossing over of senses so that a colour is heard, for example. Thoughts merge, and normal intellectual activity is suspended. The mood changes may be complex, ranging from euphoria to acute anxiety and deep depression in the course of one trip. The sensed universe and the person may seem to fragment and disintegrate, in which case friendly support is essential. Suicides and murders have unquestionably been committed during LSD trips, but there is evidence that such extreme psychotic behaviour is a reflection of the non-drugged personality and not an effect of the drug. In any event, chlorpormazine (q.v.), a barbiturate (see 'Phenobarbitone') or a tranquillizer (q.v.) can be used to end a bad trip.

LSD has been associated with the development of acute leukaemia. It has also been said to cause chromosomal damage, but the evidence indicates that damage to the genetic molecules is no more frequent when LSD is used than under normal circumstances. The drug is not known directly to cause death in man. It is not addictive, but tolerance does develop so that more of the agent is required to produce the same effects. There is cross-tolerance to mescaline and psilocybin despite the chemical differences among the three compounds.

Cannabis is hallucinogenic only with relatively high doses. In other respects, too, it differs from the amphetamine-like and indoleamine hallucinogens. In animals, cannabis has a depressant effect, like a barbiturate, and many human users say that it helps them to sleep. Yet the drug also prolongs the stimulatory activity of amphetamine. Its mode of action is believed to differ from that of the other hallucinogens, but it is not understood.

The drug, one of the oldest known to man, comes from the flowering tops and leaves of hemp, *Cannabis sativa*. The resin is called 'hashish' in North Africa, 'hash' in contemporary western societies, and 'charas' in the Orient. Resin from the small leaves and branches is 'ganja', and the dried leaves and flowers are 'bhang' or 'grass'. The word 'marijuana' applies to the whole plant or the resin, as do 'pot', 'dope' and 'shit', although the latter word probably refers originally to the colour of some hashish. The active ingredients are chemicals called cannabinols, the most active being delta 9-tetrahydrocannabinol (THC). Hashish and THC can be eaten. Hashish gives an unusual, sweetish flavour to sauces and can be baked into biscuits and pastries with no loss of activity. Cannabis is three times more potent when it is inhaled, however. On the other hand, the cannabinol content of marijuana cigarettes varies enormously from less than half a milligram of THC to more than 41 milligrams, according to one study. Both the highest and the lowest THC content were in 'joints' using 'grass'.

In the nineteenth century, cannabis was used as an anaesthetic. It has antibacterial activity, and in 1972, a report for the Canadian government stated that the drug may help to fight flu and the common cold.

After ingestion, pulse rate usually increases, blood pressure may rise slightly and urination may become more frequent. Appetite appears to grow, especially for sweets, but there are no related changes in blood-sugar content. Some users say that cannabis taken with alcohol produces severe headache. Others are not so affected, but in any event cannabis users tend not to drink when they smoke. When high doses of THC are injected into rats, foetal damage ensues. Cannabis has been shown to lead to changes in lung tissue similar to those produced by tobacco, but there is no evidence that cannabis causes lung cancer. Recent studies have shown that the ability of the heart to adapt to exercise may be diminished somewhat by cannabis. No other biophysical effects are known at present, but 'nobody can be sure that cannabis is safe in the narrow sense of pharmacology' ('Keep off the Grass', *Nature*, 221: 205, 1969).

It is not just the rigid limits of the experimental data that concern lawmakers and the scientists who advise them, however. The behavioural effects of cannabis explain both its growing popularity and the debate about its legalization. Some 20 million Americans and between two and five million Britons are said to use it with some regularity. The user may experience a dreamy, abstracted state, the slowing of time, hilarity and a heightened awareness of sound, colour and self. Sexual interest is diminished, if it is affected at all, but sensual pleasure may be much increased. Violence and aggression are very rare inasmuch as the usual high evokes reverie and relaxation. There is no evidence of long-term personality change, though psychotic reactions such as paranoia have been noted. Some tolerance to the drug may develop, but it is not addictive and there are no withdrawal symptoms. Such behavioural effects tend to be subjective and are hard to define exactly.

Objective evidence of impairment of motor tasks is lacking, except in first-time users. Experienced subjects tested with alcohol and cannabis in a driving simulator exhibited 97·44 errors under the influence of alcohol, 84·49 with cannabis and 84·46 with no drug. Nevertheless, the cannabis-induced disruption of time sense suggests that driving could be dangerous during a high.

Habitual cannabis users experience a tendency towards more free association, more vivid imagery and a temporary forgetfulness or loss of short-term memory when they are smoking. Evaluations of academic performance by cannabis users and non-users show contradictory results. The degree of memory impairment appears to depend on the assigned task, as it does in all circumstances. 'In general, the performance of experienced marijuana users on behavioural tasks is not as susceptible to the disruptive effects of marijuana as is that of drug-naïve humans even though the subjective effects of marijuana may become more intense with repeated drug experiences', according to one study (D. M. Grilly, D. P. Ferraro, R. G. Marriott, *Nature*, 242: 119–20, 1973). Some experienced users claim that they experience a memory deficit, but it is hard to obtain objective substantiation. It would seem that the more one uses marijuana, the less is the effect of the drug on behaviour and the more pleasure it affords. Perhaps both responses are psychological adjustments to the biophysical action of cannabis.

There is statistical evidence that users of heroin and other 'hard' drugs have in many cases begun their drug experiences with cannabis, but there is no way of knowing whether the use of cannabis leads on to heroin in a statistically significant number of cases. At this point, it seems reasonable to assume that there are those who will turn to hard drugs with or without a first step via cannabis.

The social implications of such questions are even less subject to statistical experimental treatment than the behavioural effects of the drug. Quite apart from what it does in the brain, cannabis use is from the psychological standpoint a kind of lotus-eating, as is the use of alcohol and nicotine. Society must decide where the individual right to opt out ends against the barbed wire of communal responsibility. It is argued that both alcohol and tobacco would be legally prohibited today had their biophysical dangers been known when use of these substances began in the distant past, but the relevance of such an historical 'if' to the present legislation on cannabis is doubtful. The United States' attempt to bar social use of alcohol (to say nothing of more recent efforts in both Britain and the United States to diminish tobacco use) failed completely. The failure was not only immediate with respect to the law – or the anti-smoking propaganda; prohibition of alcohol taught an entire generation not only that the law was something to be got round, but that laws and the institutions which make and enforce them are at best disreputable and at worst ridiculous. As the founder of behaviourism, John B. Watson, observed, 'With the successful breaking of [the prohibition law], fear of law has been removed; and when a taboo has been broken with impunity not only does that particular taboo . . . lose its grip, but all of the taboos . . . tend to become ineffective . . .' (J. B. Watson, *Behaviourism*, London: Kegan Paul, 1931, 42). Continued prohibition of cannabis reinforces the anti-social behaviour of those who use it undetected: prohibition as well as inequitable law enforcement diminish their tenuous respect for institutions which, among other serious internal contradictions, allow alcohol and tobacco despite their all too familiar dangers, and prohibit cannabis. Certainly there is a risk with this as with any drug; new evidence could demonstrate that a real danger exists. Nevertheless, in view of social attitudes towards alcohol and tobacco, and in view of the western principle of respect for the individual, a case may be made for the early legalization of cannabis.

Halothane

(Suckling, 1956, U.S.) Trade name: Fluothane. Administration: gas, often mixed with nitrous oxide (laughing gas).

Classification and therapeutic use
Developed under the aegis of the British Medical Research Council as part of a successful search for a non-explosive general anaesthetic which could be administered as a gas. Nitrous oxide, though it is not inflammable itself, can ignite when mixed with oxygen, and is difficult to control. Ether and chloroform, as well as more recent anaesthetic agents such as ethylene and cyclo-propane, are both inflammable and explosive. Halothane has been called the 'most useful general-purpose agent' in one review of anaesthetics.[*] It is non-irritating to the respiratory

[*] J. P. Payne, 'Advances in Anaesthesia', *The Practitioner*, 201:652, October 1968.

tract, and does not restrict the supply of oxygen in the mixture breathed by the patient. The compound is particularly useful for surgery on asthmatic patients because it causes expansion of the tiny tubes which conduct air within the lungs (bronchioles). Because it tends to lower blood pressure both centrally, by direct depression of heart action, and peripherally by relaxing muscles in small blood vessels, it is used for 'bloodless' plastic surgery. Because it also tends to relax the uterus, halothane can be helpful in certain difficult birth situations, though it is not employed for routine deliveries. And of course it is non-inflammable and non-explosive.

Halothane is normally employed either with oxygen alone, or with nitrous oxide-oxygen mixtures. Indeed, halothane is probably the most useful anaesthetic available today, and is likely to remain so for some time to come.

Disadvantages and side effects
Induction of anaesthesia is relatively slow, and recovery is also prolonged. The drug is not itself a pain-killer so that pethidine or an opiate (see 'Morphine') is often given first. A muscle relaxant (curare or gallamine) and a barbiturate (see 'Phenobarbitone') may also be used for premedication, depending on the type and length of the operation. Very rarely, nausea and vomiting will result from use of this agent, but the fact that its odour is not unpleasant reduces these effects. Rapid, shallow breathing can appear, at least until deep anaesthesia is achieved, at which time this effect usually disappears. However, because the drug reduces blood pressure and sensitizes heart muscle to catecholamines (see 'Adrenaline'), respiratory disturbance can presage serious slowing of the heartbeat and even cardiac arrest. These effects can be prevented by careful administration, and reversed by reduction in the amount of anaesthetic and increase in the amount of oxygen in the mixture. There is some evidence that halothane can occasionally evoke an allergy-type reaction in the liver which can damage that organ. It is thought unlikely that the drug itself is the basic cause, but such liver damage can in extreme cases be fatal. Because the anaesthetic has been blamed for foetal malformations, its use should probably be avoided during pregnancy.

Chemistry and physiology

Halothane is a simple halogenated molecule (i.e. a molecule containing chlorine, fluorine or bromine), combined with a minute amount of a stabilizing agent, thymol:

$$\begin{array}{ccc} & F & H \\ & | & | \\ F- & C-C & -Br \\ & | & | \\ & F & Cl \end{array} \qquad \text{Halothane}$$

It acts reversibly by depressing the central nervous system, first at the cerebral cortex, gradually descending to the respiratory and cardiac centres. Its molecular mechanism of action is unknown, though like other anaesthetics, it may alter the conformation of certain molecules in the membranes that surround cells, thus changing the cellular contents and activities.

The cardiovascular side effects – lowered blood pressure and the slowing of heartbeat – arise from complicated interactions of the drug, the autonomic nervous system (see 'Adrenaline') which regulates muscle both in the heart and in peripheral blood vessels, and the muscle cells themselves. This interaction is affected by the amount of the drug in the circulation, the speed of administration and of course the prior state of the patient (e.g. the strength of the heart itself).

Heparin

(Howell and Holt, 1918, U.S.) Trade names: Contusol, Hepacort Plus, Heparin Chibret, Heparin Retard, Hirudoid, Pularin; U.S.: Liquaemin Sodium. Administration: intravenous injection; topical in ointments, eye drops.

Classification
A naturally occurring substance found in human liver, lungs and heart, this anti-coagulant was discovered (McLean, 1916, U.S.) in a search for a drug which would enhance blood clotting. Although no similar compounds are known, a number of oral anti-coagulants have been synthesized during the last twenty-five years (see 'Dicoumarol').

Therapeutic uses
The major clinical use of heparin is to prevent thrombosis, that is, the blockage of a blood vessel by a thrombus, or clot, composed of blood cells and a normal blood constituent called fibrin

('Chemistry and physiology', below), which has built up at some place on the wall of the circulatory system for reasons unknown. Myocardial infarction is a form of heart attack commonly caused by the blockage of the blood vessels in heart muscle; blockage leads to death by oxygen starvation (anoxia) of those muscle cells served by the blocked vessels. If the blockage is general, or if it takes place in a major vessel leading into the heart muscle, death will quickly ensue, but this is not usually the case. The objective of anti-coagulant therapy, therefore, is to prevent formation of new thrombi which might cause additional heart attacks.

Angina pectoris is an acute, intensely painful 'heart attack' caused by anoxia or by a shortage of nutrients (ischaemia) in heart muscle. In the anginal patient, an attack can be brought on by excitement or exercise. Although the attack is not due to a thrombus, long-term treatment with anti-coagulants improves the chances of survival with this condition, presumably because the appearance of clots in tissue damaged by anoxia or ischaemia is prevented. For similar reasons, heparin and the oral anti-coagulants are used to protect patients with rheumatic heart disease associated with rheumatic fever.

Thrombosis may occur in blood vessels other than those in the heart, of course. In particular, emboli (thrombi floating in the blood, though an embolism may also be caused by fat particles or any other particulate matter or air in the blood) may block veins, where pressure is low, and pulmonary and cerebral blood vessels. This is especially true after surgery, and heparin is sometimes used to prevent post-surgical thrombo–embolism. It is also commonly employed to prevent the clotting of blood as it passes through kidney machines.

Side effects

Heparin has a low incidence of side effects, but those which occur may include allergy-type reactions such as asthma and hives, and a transient loss of hair which can occur three to four months after treatment with the agent is stopped. The chief danger is haemorrhage. No anti-coagulant should be used without careful laboratory supervision of its day-to-day effect on the blood-clotting mechanisms. Heparin ought not to be given to people with a tendency to bleed (e.g. haemophiliacs), in cases of threatened abortion, ulcers or shock, and some physicians believe that it should not be employed during pregnancy. In the event of heparin-induced haemorrhage which continues after withdrawal of the drug, one of two agents – protamine or hexadimethrine bromide (polybrine) – is usually given. Heparin acts rapidly after injection, and disappears from the blood within a few hours.

Chemistry and physiology

In contrast to the pharmacological uses of heparin ('Therapeutic uses' above), the physiological functions of this natural substance are unclear. It is believed to be one of several compounds in the body which balance the factors responsible for blood clotting (below), and may also have a secondary physiological purpose which, some believe, can be exploited therapeutically. With an enzyme (q.v.) normally present in the blood, lipoprotein lipase, heparin assists in the dispersion of fat-like molecules through capillary walls into tissue. Although prolonged administration presents difficulties, it may be preferred in treatment of heart diseases associated with thrombosis because it tends to lower the level of blood lipids (fat-like molecules). Lipids are the biochemical precursors of cholesterol which is thought to be one of the causative factors leading to atherosclerosis ('hardening of the arteries'; see 'Cholestyramine'), a condition which clearly contributes to heart disease.

Heparin is a mucopolysaccharide; that is, a series of linked sugar molecules on which amines and sulphate (SO_4) substitutions also appear. These are combined as sulphamine groups, and heparin is the strongest organic acid in the body. The substance itself has not been isolated from whole blood, and its molecular mechanism of action is unknown.

The points at which heparin interrupts the process of blood clotting are reasonably clear, however. Whole blood coagulates because a blood protein called fibrin forms a fibrous network at the site where the clot forms. Other blood elements are caught in this net. Under normal circumstances, flow stops within three to five minutes; thereafter the clot tends to become progressively harder until it is reabsorbed during healing.

Obviously, it is impossible for fibrin as such to exist in the blood. If it did, this liquid tissue would solidify. Therefore, until a circumstance such as a wound occurs, fibrin exists only as its own soluble precursor, fibrinogen. When a clot forms, another blood protein, thrombin, combines with fibrinogen and splits off a few atoms from the latter molecule to form 'fibrin monomer'. Many of these monomer units then combine (polymerize) to form a larger protein – fibrin. Like fibrin, however, thrombin cannot exist normally because if it did fibrinogen in the blood would be split immediately, forming fibrin. Once more, thrombin occurs in a precursor form, prothrombin, which is activated by another substance called thromboplastin in the presence of calcium ions (q.v.). Thromboplastin may be of two kinds, intrinsic (i.e. found in the blood) and extrinsic (found in tissue outside the bloodstream), but both appear to be necessary to convert prothrombin to thrombin.

In fact, at least seven other factors, in addition to calcium ions, are thought to participate in the formation of thromboplastin; they appear to act sequentially, just as prothrombin is converted to thrombin which splits fibrinogen with formation of fibrin.

Because each step falls away into the next, this sequence is called a cascade (see discussion of inflammation under 'Aspirin'). It is thought to look schematically like this:

(1) Factor XII → XIIa
(2)　　　　　　　XI → XIa
(3)　　　　　　　　　　IX → IXa
(4)　　　　　　　　　　　　　VIII → VIIIa
(5)　　　　　　　　　　　　　　　　X → Xa
(6)　　　　　　　　　　　　　　　　　　　V → Va
(7)　　　　　　　　　　　Prothrombin → Thrombin
(8)　　　　　　　　　　　Fibrinogen → Fibrin

Bell, Davidson and Scarborough, *op cit.*, p. 451

In addition, a factor XIII normally exists to stabilize the clot. Haemophilia is usually caused by the congenital absence of either factor VIII or factor IX.

Heparin acts at three points at least. It interferes with the formation of thromboplastin (the exact method of interference is not clear), it inhibits formation of thrombin from prothrombin, and the binding of thrombin to fibrinogen.

Hormone

(Greek: *hormon* – impelling)

Hormones are chemical substances which are secreted into the bloodstream and which act on cells elsewhere in the body to produce an effect. They may be steroid (below) or polypeptide (see 'Biochemistry') in nature. More recently the use of the term has been expanded to include substances, which may be simpler compounds, produced in tissues (for example, nerve endings) and which act close to their site of origin. These are referred to as 'local hormones', and will be discussed at the end of this entry.

The glands in the body which produce hormones are known collectively as the endocrine system, and include the pituitary or hypophysis, the adrenals, the gonads – ovary in the female, testis in the male – the thyroid, the parathyroids and the Islets of Langerhans in the pancreas (see 'Insulin').

Pituitary

The pituitary is a small pea-shaped gland located in the centre of the skull immediately under a part of the brain known as the hypothalamus. Until recently it was thought that the pituitary controlled the entire endocrine system, the 'conductor of the endocrine orchestra' so to speak. However, recently it has been shown that it is itself controlled by nervous impulses from the adjacent hypothalamus (to the posterior part of the pituitary) and by a special modification of the blood vessels in that area – the hypophyseal portal system – which picks up polypeptide 're-leasing factors' produced in nerve cells of the hypothalamus, and carries them to the anterior part of the pituitary where they cause cells to secrete hormones.

The pituitary, in man, is divided into two lobes, anterior – the adenohypophysis, and posterior – the neurohypophysis. In lower animals an intermediate lobe, which secretes a hormone known as MSH or melanocyte-stimulating hormone concerned with pigmentation, is present. In man it is uncertain whether MSH is produced as a separate entity, the picture being further complicated by the fact that another anterior pituitary hormone – ACTH – can have similar activity. Certainly what intermediate tissue is present is poorly developed and absorbed into the anterior lobe.

The *posterior pituitary* has nervous connexions with the adjacent hypothalamus which control its secretion of two hormones – antidiuretic hormone (ADH, also known as vasopressin) and oxytocin. It is thought that these substances are not actually produced in the posterior pituitary but travel there down the nerve fibres which connect it to the hypothalamus, the hormones having been synthesized in special collections of nerve cells known as the supra-optic and paraventricular nuclei. Both ADH and oxytocin have been identified as nonapeptides (that is peptides with nine amino acids).

ADH in small physiological doses decreases the amount of water excreted in the urine, possibly by increasing the size of the pores in the cells lining the distal tubule in the kidney (see 'Diuretic'). In larger doses it raises the blood pressure by causing capillary constriction, which is why it was originally named 'vasopressin'. The secretion of ADH is controlled mainly by the osmotic pressure of the blood plasma due to its electrolyte (q.v.) content, an increase in which causes increased secretion of ADH to retain water and dilute the plasma electrolytes back down to their normal concentration. The reverse is also seen. The nerve cells which mediate these changes are called osmoreceptors (i.e. receptors sensitive to osmotic pressure), and lie near the supra-optic nucleus in the brain. A direct effect on ADH secretion may occur in states of anger or fear where nervous hypothalamic stimulation could explain the decreased urine *formation* which occurs. Indeed, the higher ADH production under these conditions may partly explain the increase in blood pressure (vasopressin activity) and pallor (capillary constriction) which characterize these emotions.

Oxytocin stimulates a type of muscle known as smooth muscle which is present in the body in various sites, including the secretory tissues of the breast, the gut and the uterus. Thus it aids childbirth (uterine muscle), the ejection of milk from the breast and in high doses it may cause a slight fall in blood pressure due to a relaxing effect on the smooth muscle of blood vessels.

Synthetic forms of both oxytocin and vasopressin are available and in the future may well replace extracts of posterior pituitary, now more frequently used. Oxytocin is used for induction of labour, to stimulate the 'lazy uterus' during labour, to cause uterine contraction either after surgery or to control bleeding after childbirth and to stimulate milk ejection during breast feeding if the breast becomes engorged. Vasopressin is used to control surgical shock (by producing capillary contraction), and in the treatment of diabetes insipidus (see 'Chlorothiazide') a condition characterized by deficient secretion of ADH by the neurohypophysis, possibly due to compression by a tumour of the anterior pituitary, or to destruction following a small clot which cuts off the supply of blood to the gland. Due to the deficiency of ADH the patient excretes large amounts of very dilute urine and consequently consumes large quantities of water. Posterior pituitary extract either as an injection or in the form of nasal snuff controls the diuresis.

The *anterior pituitary* has no nervous connexion with the hypothalamus, and depends for its control on two interconnected mechanisms. The first of these is the hypophyseal portal system (above) which also acts as part of the second, the aptly named 'feedback mechanism'. Each of the anterior pituitary hormones (with the possible exception of STH and Prolactin below) acts on a specific endocrine organ to cause it to secrete specific hormones into the bloodstream. In order that reasonably constant levels of these hormones can be maintained in the bloodstream it is necessary that some mechanism exist whereby the stimulating (or 'trophic') hormone produced by the pituitary may be switched off. This is the feedback mechanism which consists of cells in the hypothalamus, and possibly the pituitary also, which are sensitive to the level of hormone circulating in the blood, and which switch off the production of either releasing factors (hypothalamus) or trophic hormones (pituitary) when the level rises above the threshold. When the 'switch-off' has operated, the specific endocrine organ ceases to produce hormone, and the circulating level falls again. When it falls below the threshold, the production of releasing factors and trophic hormones recommences, thus restimulating the specific endocrine organ. Each endocrine organ has an independent negative feedback loop which is in general not affected by changes in the circulating levels of hormones other than those produced by itself.

The following hormones are produced by the anterior pituitary – growth hormone, or somatrophin (STH); adrenocorticotrophic hormone (ACTH), which in man is closely related to melanocyte-stimulating hormone; thyrotrophic hormone (TSH); follicle-stimulating hormone (FSH); luteinizing hormone (LH) which is produced in the female and is identical to interstitial-cell-stimulating hormone (ICSH) in the male; and prolactin, which is also called lactogenic hormone or mammotrophin.

As its name suggests, *growth hormone* (somatrophin, STH) is necessary for normal growth. Should its production become deficient due to disease, growth becomes stunted, and dwarfism occurs. Excessive production of hormone, however, causes either giantism if the long bones of the body have not ceased growing, or if they have, acromegaly in which there is enlargement of the lower half of the face, the hands and the feet.

Growth hormone is a protein. Neither its structure nor its cellular mode of action is certain, but at the tissue level it promotes retention in the body of nitrogen, calcium, phosphorus, potassium and sodium. As might be expected, therefore, administration of the compound causes increased growth and deposition of bone (calcium and phosphorus), and increased formation of protein (nitrogen) both in skeletal muscles and in the liver. The increased protein formation is caused partly by diversion of amino acids from synthesis of the metabolic waste product, urea; where the circulating level of urea is elevated due to kidney failure, STH may be used to reduce it towards normal. Increased protein formation is also due to an acceleration of amino-acid transport into the cells. It is possible that this latter effect may require the presence of insulin (q.v.).

Growth hormone and insulin normally have antagonistic actions, however, designed to keep the supply of energy-yielding substances in the blood fairly constant. Thus shortly after a meal the blood level of insulin is high and causes deposition of glucose into fat and tissue protein, and at this time the level of growth hormone is low. Later, as the blood glucose level drops, the secretion of growth hormone increases and it acts with insulin as described above to promote protein synthesis. Still later, however, as the blood glucose becomes rather low, growth hormone secretion increases considerably and deposited fat is now drawn on to provide energy sources. If the normal control of growth hormone secretion is lost due, for example, to excessive production, a condition resembling diabetes mellitus (see 'Insulin') may be produced and may be accentuated by damage to the Islet cells (below) which produce insulin; it is noteworthy that diabetes mellitus is a not uncommon accompaniment of acromegaly.

Adrenocorticotrophic hormone (ACTH) acts on the outer part of the adrenal gland (below) and stimulates the production of corticosteroids (see 'Hydrocortisone'). Possibly due to the fact that the adrenal was one of the earliest of the endocrine glands to engage the attention of physiologists (the first description of the disease resulting from their destruction appeared in 1855

(Addison)) more is known about ACTH than about any of the other anterior pituitary hormones.

ACTH is a polypeptide whose structure differs in different species. However, all species studied to date exhibit the same sequence of amino acids from number 1 to number 24, differences being found in sequence 25 to 33 of the full thirty-nine amino acids. It is of interest that a synthetic compound with the correct sequence of 1 to 24 has been found to have full biological activity, and, indeed, such a preparation is currently available.

The production of ACTH from the pituitary is under two forms of control: a negative feedback effected by the circulating level of corticosteroid, and a stimulating control via the hypothalamus mediated by the corticotrophin-releasing factor, which responds to stress, either within the body (for example, severe decrease in blood sugar) or from without (for example, severe cold or burns). It is possible that the stress reaction is associated with the emotional rather than the strictly physical content of the experience. For example, one of the highest ever plasma ACTH levels recorded was in a medical student who, subsequent to being given two millilitres of normal saline intravenously, was told that the experimenting doctor had made a mistake and given him a dose of insulin sufficient to kill him. The saline would have produced no effect, but the emotional shock certainly did!

At its target organ – the adrenal cortex – ACTH causes an immediate discharge of stored steroid (below) and stimulates further synthesis. Initially it appears to stimulate the conversion of ATP (see 'Biochemistry') to a compound known as $3',5'$-adenosine monophosphate cyclic ester ($3',5'$-AMP) which activates an enzyme (q.v.), phosphorylase. The enzyme increases the catabolism of glycogen to glucose-6-phosphate. In addition ACTH stimulates the transport of glucose into the cell (with subsequent conversion to glucose-6-phosphate). This compound is then broken down through a pathway of metabolism which produces $NADPH_2$ (reduced nucleotide adenine diphosphate, see 'Vitamin'), which may be regarded as an energy store in the cell, and which is subsequently utilized for further production of steroid.

ACTH also helps to maintain an adequate supply of steroid to the body by decreasing the rate at which the main circulating steroid (hydrocortisone, q.v.) is broken down (or deactivated) in the liver. Thus the steroid, once produced, circulates in the body for a longer period of time and is available to enable the body to respond to the precipitating stress.

The therapeutic uses of ACTH, either synthetic or purified extracts of animal pituitaries, are all mediated through the final common pathway of increased steroid production from the adrenal cortex, and indeed it has been suggested by some authors that 'there is no substantial evidence that any therapeutic goals can be attained with ACTH that cannot be attained with appropriate doses of currently available steroids'.* There is one use for ACTH, however, which is of paramount importance: it is a diagnostic aid in adrenal deficiency. In the normal patient the injection of ACTH is followed by a rapid rise in the circulating hydrocortisone level. In the patient with non-functioning adrenals, no such rise occurs.

Thyroid-stimulating hormone (TSH) acts on the thyroid gland (see below, and 'Methimazole') to stimulate the output of thyroid hormone. It stimulates the uptake of oxygen and the use of glucose by the cells of the thyroid gland in tissue culture. The increased output of thyroid hormone from the gland which follows the administration of TSH is thought to be a result of the stimulated metabolism of the thyroid cells with subsequent activation of enzymes (q.v.) which split the thyroid hormone from protein to which it is normally bound for storage.

The control of TSH output from the anterior pituitary is subject to two influences: the negative feedback previously described in relation to ACTH, the response in this case being to the circulating level of thyroid hormone which influences both hypothalamic receptors and the anterior pituitary cells direct; and, independent of the feedback mechanism, to the hypothalamic sensitivity to temperature and possibly stress. Thus exposure to cold is accompanied by increased release of TSH with consequent increased release of thyroid hormone to stimulate the body's metabolism and restore its temperature to normal.

TSH has been isolated in a pure form from anterior pituitary extracts, and found to be a glyco-protein (that is, a chemical combination of amino acids and compounds related to glucose). It is not used medically in treatment of thyroid disease, but it can be used for diagnosis because it distinguishes between the decreased function due to primary disease of the thyroid gland and that due to decreased function of the anterior pituitary.

Follicle-stimulating hormone (FSH), like TSH, is a

* Goodman and Gilman, *op. cit.*, p. 1614.

glycoprotein. It is one of the group of hormones known as gonadotrophin (that is, hormones which stimulate the gonads, or reproductive organs) which also includes LH (or ICSH) and prolactin, produced in the anterior pituitary (as is FSH), and human chorionic gonadotrophin and pregnant mare serum gonadotrophin (below) produced in the placenta (or after-birth). With the exception of prolactin, a simple protein, all of these substances are glyco-proteins.

FSH secretion is thought to be mediated entirely through the hypothalamus which produces FSH-releasing factor. The release of this substance is subject to a negative feedback mediated by the circulating level of oestrogen (q.v.) and also to a positive stimulus of light (rats exposed to constant illumination go into a condition known as constant oestrus which is thought to be due to continual oestrogenic stimulation induced by continuous FSH release). FSH production in the female varies cyclically during the menstrual cycle, being high during the first fourteen days and subsequently decreasing as the circulating level of oestrogen, whose production in the ovary it has stimulated (below), rises. At menopause, when ovarian function and the production of oestrogen declines, very high levels of FSH may be produced. They are thought to be responsible for the occurrence of 'hot flushes'. Administration of oestrogen-containing preparations at this time is extremely effective in controlling these symptoms, presumably by decreasing the pituitary production of FSH via the feedback mechanism.

In the male the function of FSH is less clear. Originally it was thought that it stimulated the production of spermatozoa ('Testis', below), but recent evidence in animals has shown that the administration of pure FSH to males from whom the pituitary had been removed is ineffective in stimulating this process. However, addition of small amounts of ICSH(LH) caused spermatogenesis to recommence. Thus FSH in the male appears to be an accessory factor, rather than primarily responsible.

Little is known about the mechanism of action of FSH at the cellular level.

Production of *luteinizing hormone* (LH) is subject to the stimulation of LH-releasing factor from the hypothalamus. A negative feedback mechanism controlling LH-releasing factor and responding to the circulating level of progesterone (q.v.) is present; in addition, the hypothalamic release of this compound appears to be stimulated by certain visual stimuli (at least in birds which will not ovulate if caged alone but will commence egg production, presumably due to LH release, in response to the presence of another bird, or even their own reflection in a mirror) and possibly by intercourse (at least in rabbits).

LH production in the human female is largely localized to the period of mid-cycle when, in response to a rising level of circulating oestrogen in the blood, a sudden release of LH (presumably preceded by a surge of LH-releasing factor from the hypothalamus) occurs and triggers off the release of an ovum in the ovary. Subsequent to this release LH acts on the tissue left behind in the ovary (below) producing changes which result in the production of progesterone; this in turn causes the secretion of LH to be diminished via negative feedback.

In the male LH or rather *interstitial-cell-stimulating hormone* (ICSH) which is the same substance under another name, stimulates the cells of the testis (below) which produce the main male hormone – testosterone. This compound, which is responsible for the male sexual characteristics and which stimulates spermatogenesis, operates the feedback mechanism to the hypothalamus, and thus controls the secretion of ICSH in the male.

The existence of *prolactin* in humans is not absolutely established. Preparations of human growth hormone have some prolactin-like activity which may, of course, reflect incomplete separation rather than chemical identity. It is particularly involved in breast development and lactation. In a breast which has been stimulated by oestrogen and progesterone, for example in later pregnancy, it causes increase in the growth of the milk-secreting tissue. After the birth of the child the circulating level of oestrogen stimulates the production of prolactin by the pituitary, and this in its turn stimulates the initiation of lactation. Higher levels of oestrogen, however, such as may be administered medically, can inhibit lactation after childbirth, presumably diminishing the secretion of prolactin.

The so-called 'fertility drugs' for the treatment of human infertility are, with one exception, preparations of gonadotrophins. Of these, two are commercially available, while a third is used in specialized obstetric and gynaecological clinics. The two available preparations are human chorionic gonadotrophin (HCG) which is concentrated from the urine of pregnant women in whom it is formed in the placenta, and is a glyco-protein similar in action, although not entirely in chemical structure, to LH. It also has definite luteotrophic activity (that is, it stimulates the activity of the corpus luteum. 'Ovary', below). It is used to induce ovulation subsequent to a course of pretreatment with an FSH type of preparation. Such a preparation is pregnant mare serum gonadotrophin, which is prepared by purification from the blood serum of pregnant mares. It acts mainly like FSH and produces development of follicles in the ovary. Ovulation may occur if the LH content is sufficiently high or, if not, it can be produced by an injection of HCG.

The third preparation which is used only in special clinics, because of the extreme care required in controlling the dosage, is prepared from human post-menopausal urine, and has largely FSH activity. It is called Pergonal, and is commonly used to induce enlargement in the ovary, of the egg and its surrounding tissues, treatment being followed by the injection of HCG to induce ovulation.

The fourth preparation used to treat infertility – clomiphene – is not a gonadotrophin at all. When given to human patients, clomiphene produces considerable enlargement of the ovaries, and ovulation has been induced in a significant number of infertile cases. The compound is anti-oestrogenic, and appears to act by stimulating the production of gonadotrophins from the pituitary, possibly by blocking the normal feedback inhibition by oestrogen. The indications to date are that the secretion of both FSH and LH is stimulated.

Much publicity surrounded some of the early results of the use of these four compounds, not altogether surprising in view of the multiple pregnancies which frequently resulted. In addition emergency admissions to hospital occurred due to excessive stimulation and enlargement of the ovaries. Almost without exception it is safe to say that these effects were a result of overdosage in the early days of use of the drugs; with the introduction of modern laboratory technology allowing precise control of the degree of ovarian stimulation, they may be expected to contribute both significantly and safely to the control of fertility, or rather infertility. Their use is being investigated for treatment of male infertility, and of a condition known as undescended testis, where one of the testes remains in the abdominal cavity rather than descending into the scrotum.

The *peripheral endocrine glands* are the thyroid, the parathyroids, the Islets of the pancreas, the adrenals, ovaries in the female and testes in the male. These are of varying importance in controlling the functions of the body, although of them the adrenal is probably the most vital.

The *thyroid* gland lies in the neck and consists of two lobes lying one on either side of the windpipe joined across the front by a band of thyroid tissue known as the isthmus. Its function is controlled by secretion of TSH (above) from the pituitary. It secretes a hormone, either thyroxin or tri-iodothyronine (or both), which is primarily concerned in controlling the metabolism of the body.

For the synthesis of its hormone(s) the thyroid gland requires iodine which it obtains from circulating iodine absorbed from food. In its absence the thyroid grows bigger, producing more and larger cells, in an attempt to increase its efficiency in trapping iodine, and the condition known as goitre results. Goitre used to be quite common in certain areas of Britain where the local water supply is deficient in iodine, and this gave rise to the old name for goitre – 'Derbyshire neck'. To combat the condition, iodine is now added to table salt.

From the trapped iodine and the amino acid tyrosine the thyroid first manufactures thyroxin:

$$HO-\underset{I}{\overset{I}{\underset{}{\bigcirc}}}-O-\underset{I}{\overset{I}{\underset{}{\bigcirc}}}-CH_2 \cdot CH(NH_2)COOH$$

This, the thyroid hormone, is normally stored in the follicle bound to complex proteins until it is required in the body, when, under the influence of the enzyme, protease, it is split off from these and released into the bloodstream.

Thyroxin, and its related compound tri-iodothyronine, which lacks one iodine atom, have a wide variety of metabolic stimulant effects in the body. They stimulate the uptake of oxygen and production of heat by the tissues, increase the heart rate, blood pressure, skin circulation (to get rid of the excess heat), muscle activity and activity of the nervous system, the growth and development of tissues such as the gonads and bones (although excess production can lead to loss of bone substance with weakening of the long bones) and help to maintain milk production during lactation.

Their stimulatory effects may occur because thyroid hormone enhances reactions within intra-cellular organelles known as mitochondria – the 'power-houses' of the cell – whose numbers per cell have been shown to be increased in hyperthyroid animals, and which become more porous after administration of thyroid hormone. The rise in oxygen utilization and heat production could be explained by a partial uncoupling of oxidative phosphorylation (see discussion under 'Vitamin', and 'Aspirin') so that more oxidative metabolism (and therefore oxygen uptake and heat production) is required to produce an equivalent amount of ATP.

Hyperthyroidism (overactivity of the thyroid) is characterized by the nervous, irritable patient who shows all the signs of excess of circulating thyroid hormone described above. The condition is generally treated by surgical removal of three-quarters of the thyroid gland (removal of less will generally not cure the condition!) but anti-thyroid drugs are also used (see 'Methimazole').

Hypothyroidism (underactivity of the thyroid) is characterized by the physically and mentally slow, lethargic, cold patient. Treatment in these cases is either with thyroid hormone, purified extracts of animal thyroid glands or with the sodium salt of tri-iodothyronine, which is more active, although at the cellular level there appears to be no difference between the two compounds.

Immediately behind the thyroid gland lie four small yellowish masses of tissue, the *parathyroid glands*. They secrete a hormone, parathyroid hormone, which is largely responsible for maintaining the level of calcium constant in the bloodstream (see 'Vitamin', especially Vitamin D). Calcium, in association with phosphate ions, forms the hard part of bone. In addition, a certain level is required in the blood to allow the nervous system to operate properly. The hormone is a polypeptide whose structure is not completely known.

Somewhat surprisingly the secretion of parathyroid hormone does not appear to be under the control of the pituitary gland, despite the role of the latter in regulating the endocrine system. The level of parathyroid hormone is controlled directly by the blood–calcium level; a fall in blood calcium stimulates its production. It then raises the blood calcium to normal levels by increasing the reabsorption of calcium in the kidney tubule (see 'Diuretic'), the reabsorption of calcium from bone (bone is always in a dynamic state, being reabsorbed from one side while deposition of fresh bone goes on at the other), and also, possibly, by increasing the absorption of calcium from food in the gut. The increased blood-calcium level produced by all of these processes acts back on the parathyroid gland and switches off parathyroid hormone production. Thus, like all of the glands of the endocrine system, the parathyroids operate a feedback mechanism with the differences that the active principle is the blood calcium, rather than the hormone, and the site is the gland itself, rather than the hypothalamic overlord.

Calcium metabolism is directly related to the use of phosphate by the body, in part because bone is largely a compound of the two, calcium phosphate. Thus, parathyroid hormone also regulates phosphate metabolism.

The mechanism whereby parathyroid hormone causes increased bone reabsorption is not altogether clear. However, much of the evidence suggests that the hormone causes the development of osteoclasts (cells which destroy bone). It may also affect the mitochondria in these cells in combination with vitamin D (q.v.) so that a localized increase occurs in the acidity of the tissues surrounding the cells. This acidity, in its turn, dissolves the hydroxyapatite, mainly calcium phosphate, and the calcium and phosphate pass into the bloodstream.

Overactivity of the parathyroid glands, which may be due to overgrowth or occasionally a tumour, may only appear as a renal stone due to the excess of calcium excreted in the urine. However, if the disease progresses far enough, damage to the kidney tubules with a consequent loss of the ability to reabsorb water may occur and show itself as thirst, dehydration and increased urine volume. In addition weakness, loss of muscle tone, vomiting and mental symptoms are seen, and fractures may occur due to the excess reabsorption of bone.

The treatment of hyperparathyroidism is by removal of the glands or tumour. In an attempt to prevent the onset of hypoparathyroidism it is usual to leave behind a little gland tissue.

Hypoparathyroidism is much more dramatic in its clinical picture. Symptoms are mainly due to increased excitability of the nerves because of the calcium deficiency. The patient develops tetany with generalized convulsions, including contraction of the muscles which close the larynx (the entry to the windpipe) and incipient suffocation. In addition, because of the increased excitability of the sympathetic and parasympathetic nervous system (see 'Adrenaline') colic of the gut, contraction of the air passages and profuse sweating are seen.

Treatment of tetany consists of the administration of parathyroid hormone (which is extracted from bovine parathyroid glands), calcium and vitamin D. Because the parathyroid hormone causes increased reabsorption of bone, it is only used until the tetany is brought under control. Thereafter the level of plasma calcium is maintained by the addition of large quantities of calcium to the diet, and the administration of vitamin D to aid its absorption and subsequent utilization.

The pancreas itself is an exocrine gland; that is, it secretes via a duct externally in the sense that the interior of the intestine is outside the body. Note that substances secreted via a duct are not hormones according to the definition of the word with which this entry begins. Yet curiously, within the pancreas are clumps of cells, the Islets of Langerhans, which are endocrine glands. Their activity appears to be controlled by a feedback mechanism acting via routes other than the hypothalamus, at least in part. The Islets of Langerhans secrete insulin and glucagon. This tissue, which consists of multiple little clumps of cells richly supplied with blood vessels, contains two types of cells, called alpha and beta cells.

The alpha cells produce a substance known as glucagon which is a polypeptide with twenty-nine amino acids. Glucagon is secreted in response to a decrease in the blood sugar, and possibly under the stimulation of pituitary STH. It acts solely in the liver where it increases the synthesis of adenosine-3',5'-monophosphate (ACTH, above). Whether glucagon is normally active in the body is uncertain. It is available commercially as an injection in the United States for the treatment of coma due to insulin overdosage, but not in the United Kingdom. In view of the fact that insulin overdose can be treated with intravenous glucose, that glucagon requires the presence of glycogen in the liver to reverse the coma, and that irreversible brain damage can be produced by prolonged low blood-sugar levels, it should be used with caution.

The beta cells of the Islets produce insulin (q.v.), the level of secretion being regulated by the circulating glucose concentration. An increase in glucose causes higher insulin output, with consequent metabolic actions described under 'Insulin'. The effect of insulin is antagonized by growth hormone (above), by hormones from the adrenal cortex (below) and by adrenaline and glucagon.

The three remaining endocrine glands are the *adrenals*, the *ovaries* in the female and the *testes* in the male. The adrenal is really two endocrine glands in one; its central part or medulla produces adrenaline (q.v.) and noradrenaline, the former in man composing about eighty per cent of the adrenal medullary hormone content. Noradrenaline will be considered below (under local hormones), although it has some general activity in the body also.

The adrenal cortex, ovaries and testes all produce hormones which are called steroids and which have, as the central part of their molecule, the following compound:

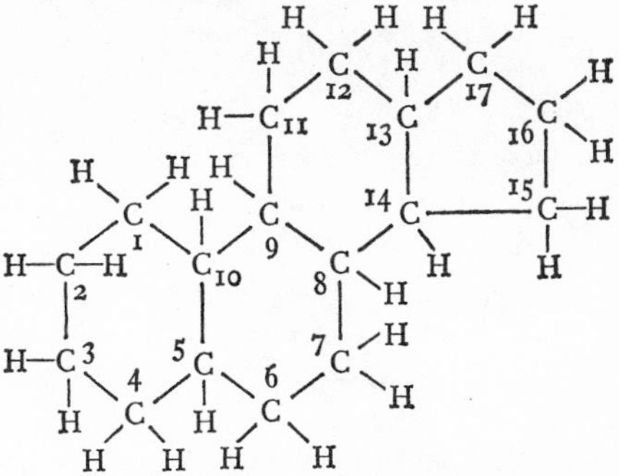

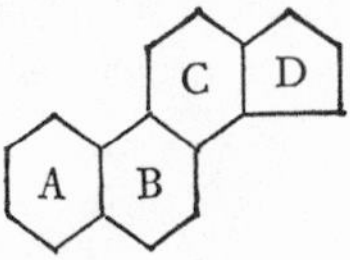

Short form of formula with ring identification (not normally inserted).

This compound is called the perhydrocyclopentenophenanthrene ring and the biological activity of individual steroid hormones depends on the chemical groups (or substitutions) on this molecule. Each carbon atom of the molecule is numbered as shown above. The numbers enable chemists to describe quickly and easily the structure of any compound under consideration. In addition, the four rings are lettered as indicated.

Four main groups of steroid hormones can be distinguished, depending on the nature of the substitutions on the central molecule. These are the oestrogens (q.v.) which have an extra methyl group (CH_3) substituted for the hydrogen on carbon 13 and numbered 18; thus the oestrogens are sometimes loosely referred to as C_{18} steroids. In addition, they have, generally, a totally unsaturated A-ring (that is, the A-ring of the molecule has three double bonds (see 'Biochemistry')) alternating with three single bonds). Various other substitutions are made on the molecule which distinguish the different oestrogens from each other. The structure of the most biologically active oestrogen in the female body, oestradiol, is shown below:

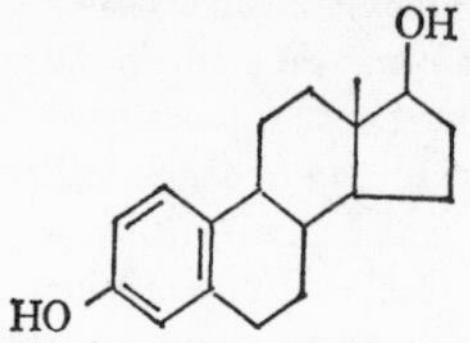

The second main group of steroid hormones is the androgens (or male hormones). In addition to a methyl group labelled number 18, these compounds have another methyl substitution for hydrogen, this time on carbon 10 and labelled carbon 19. Thus, androgens are sometimes loosely referred to as C_{19} steroids. In addition, their A-ring is only partially unsaturated and has, generally, one double bond between carbons 4 and 5. The structure of the most active male hormone, testosterone (q.v.), is shown below:

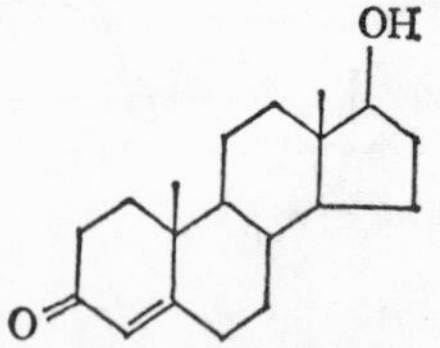

The third group of steroid hormones is the progestogens. In addition to methyl groups labelled 18 and 19, these compounds have a further substitution on carbon 17, consisting of the following group –CO–CH$_3$. The carbon atoms of this substitution are labelled 20 and 21 for the –CO and CH$_3$ respectively. Progestogens are sometimes, but not commonly, referred to as C_{21} steroids. Like testosterone, they generally have a partially unsaturated A-ring. The structure of the most active naturally occurring progestogen, progesterone (q.v.), is shown below:

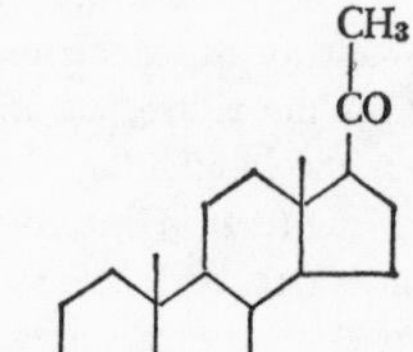

The fourth and final main group of steroid hormones is the corticosteroids. These are very similar to the progestogens in structure, except that at carbon 21 they have a $-CH_2OH$ group rather than the $-CH_3$ group of progesterone. In addition, they frequently have a substitution on carbon 11 which consists of either a hydroxyl ($-OH$) or a ketone ($=O$) group, but this is not always present (see deoxycorticosterone–DOC– under 'Hydrocortisone').

Hydrocortisone (q.v.), a typical example of the corticosteroids, is shown below:

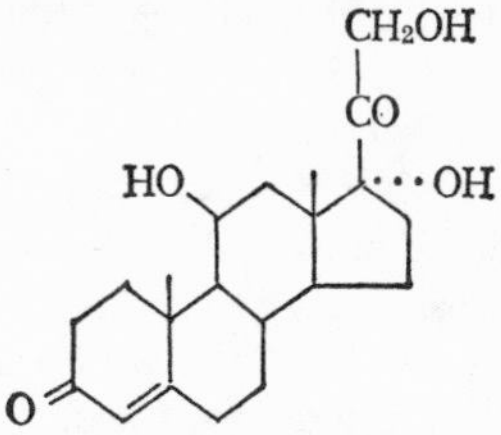

The *adrenals* are two endocrine glands, each shaped rather like a cocked hat, lying behind the back of the abdominal cavity, one on either side, on top of the kidneys. Their outer part (the cortex) produces corticosteroids, an androgen – dehydroepiandrosterone (see 'Testosterone'), a progestogen – progesterone (q.v.) and an oestrogen – oestradiol (see 'Oestrogen').

The secretion of adrenal steroids appears to be largely under the control of ACTH. Secretion of ACTH and in consequence of corticosteroids (the latter, of course, exerting a negative feedback control on the hypothalamus) does not appear to continue at the same level throughout the day. It is greatest in the early hours of the morning and declines throughout the day. This regular rhythm (the circadian rhythm) develops gradually after birth and may be related to the light–dark cycle to which we are all exposed. It appears to be remarkably firmly entrenched in our physiological make-up once it develops, but can be altered under experimental conditions. For example, volunteers living in total darkness in caves with no temporal clues become desynchronized. They develop a 'free-running' rhythm which may vary significantly from the normal twenty-four-hour cycle. Sailors on board submarines operating on a four-hours darkness, eight-hours light rhythm develop a double peak of circulating corticosteroid in twenty-four hours.

There appears to be some relationship between the level of corticosteroid in the blood and the subsequent level of mental activity about four to eight hours later. Thus, for example, the early morning peak of plasma hydrocortisone appears to be an arousal mechanism and to be followed, at a suitable interval thereafter, by wakening. Most of us know that our best period for mental activity is between nine and eleven in the morning (that is about four to six hours after the peak of plasma hydrocortisone). The desynchronization of this rhythm which occurs in air travellers may partially explain the mental inco-ordination so commonly observed after landing (and which, regrettably, is not taken into account by politicians flying from one country to another to make major policy decisions).

The control of the adrenal cortical secretion may not be altogether under the influence of ACTH. Recent work has suggested that the adrenal androgen secretion, at least, is regulated by the level of pituitary LH. Circumstantial evidence pointing to this association is seen in the observation that female patients with hirsutism (growth of beard or moustache), which many believe to be due to an excess of circulating adrenal androgen, may often have their symptoms controlled by oral contraceptives which inhibit LH production.

The adrenal cortex is vital to the body's reaction to stress (see 'Adrenaline'); a massive increase in the circulating level of plasma hydrocortisone (cortisol) assists the body in resisting the effects of such traumata as surgical operation, haemorrhage, etc. In the rare patient whose adrenals do not react to stress, sudden collapse may occur under these conditions with shock, fall in blood pressure, muscle weakness and disturbed kidney function.

Chronic adrenal insufficiency may occur, either due to destruction of the adrenal cortex (Addison's disease, p. 122, above) or to failure of the anterior pituitary cells which produce ACTH. Without ACTH secretion of corticosteroids (with the exception of aldosterone) is markedly deficient. A third type of adrenal cortical deficiency is 'congenital adrenal hyperplasia (virilism)' in which the metabolic pathways responsible for steroid production are disturbed and the adrenal produces large quantities of androgens and decreased quantities of corticosteroids. Because of decreased corticosteroid production, the feedback mechanism causes increased ACTH production and the adrenals become over-enlarged (hyperplastic). This disease, like Addison's disease, can be controlled by the administration of corticosteroids, either by mouth or by injection. The biological actions of preparations which may be used are considered under 'Hydrocortisone'.

Overactivity of the adrenal cortex results in one of three main clinical syndromes. These are *Cushing's syndrome*, due to excess production of cortisol from an adrenal tumour or hyperplastic adrenals, which is commonly associated with the presence of tumours in the anterior pituitary; the adreno-genital syndrome in which excess of androgens are produced leading to virilism in females or very occasionally excess of oestrogens with feminization in males; or *hyperaldosteronism* which is characterized by excess of production of aldosterone.

Oestrogens (q.v.) and progesterone (q.v.) are produced in the *ovaries* which are found in the female, one on either side of the lowest part of the abdominal cavity, within the bony pelvis. Each ovary consists of supporting tissue containing in its substance 100,000 to 200,000 ova, each surrounded by one or two flattened cells, these structures being known as 'primordial follicles'. Each month, two to three days after the onset of the menstrual flow and in response to an outpouring of FSH from the pituitary, about one hundred follicles start to grow and to accumulate more cells around themselves. The follicular cells secrete oestrogen in ever-increasing amounts during the first half of the cycle (causing a decrease in the amount of FSH produced due to the negative feedback mechanism) until, around day 14, release of LH from the anterior pituitary is triggered off. When this occurs the hollow follicle ruptures, the ovum is released and passes into the genital tract where it may be fertilized. The follicular cells left behind undergo a transformation, becoming enlarged and laden with fatty substances which imparts to them a yellowish colour. The resultant mass of tissue is thus called a corpus luteum (yellow body). Its cells are changed not only anatomically but also biochemically; from day 15 on they begin to secrete not only oestrogen but also increasing quantities of progesterone which is required to prepare the lining of the womb for implantation of a fertilized ovum. Should implantation not occur, the secretory function of the corpus luteum diminishes apparently sharply around day 26, and the resulting withdrawal of hormonal support causes the lining of the womb to disintegrate and to shed as the menstrual flow. Thereafter the whole process recommences.

Unlike the female, the male only produces one main gonadal hormone, testosterone. It is produced in the *testes* which can be considered anatomically to consist of two parts, a non-endocrine one, the spermatogenic tubules, which produce the spermatozoa, and an endocrine one, the interstitial cells, which lie in the spaces between the tubules. These increase in number at puberty, remain approximately constant during active sexual life and diminish in number in old age. In response to ICSH from the anterior pituitary, they secrete testosterone (q.v.), the level of secretion of which appears to be reasonably constant, rather than cyclic as in the case of oestrogens in the female. Present evidence leaves some doubt regarding the importance of testosterone in the feedback mechanism.

Local hormones

The term 'local hormones' has wide application in the physiological world. Strictly it should be applied only to substances produced at a specific tissue site and acting in the immediate neighbourhood as, for example, acetylcholine which is produced by certain nerve-endings and transmits nervous impulses to the immediately adjacent muscle or gland cell (see 'Atropine') or the other main neurotransmitter, noradrenaline (see 'Adrenaline', 'Guanethidine', 'Methyldopa', 'Phentolamine' and 'Propranolol') which acts over a similar distance.

The term is also applied to hormones derived from blood: angiotensin, which stimulates smooth muscle and raises the blood pressure, bradykinin and kallidin, which are often classed together as the plasma (blood with the formed elements removed) kinins and which also act on smooth muscle to cause dilation of blood vessels followed by a fall in blood pressure, and also stimulate pain nerve endings. 5-Hydroxytryptamine (see 'Phenelzine') is stored in the blood platelets and may be released as a 'local hormone' in response to injury or inflammation, although it is present in the brain also as a 'true' local hormone (discussed below).

Extension of the use of the term has led to its application to substances which act at a site more distant from the source of biosynthesis, like a true hormone. For example there are a number of substances produced by the gut which alter the activity of associated glands and other structures: cholecystokinin, which is produced by the duodenum and stimulates the gall-bladder to discharge bile to aid in digestion, or pancreozymin, again from the duodenum which increases the output of enzymes (q.v.) from the pancreas for similar purposes.

The 'true' local hormones are acetylcholine, catecholamines (see 'Adrenaline' and 'Amphetamine'), heparin (q.v.), histamine (see 'Tripelennamine'), 5-hydroxytryptamine (possibly the most important from a pharmacological point of view), substance P – a polypeptide (see 'Biochemistry') found chiefly in the intestine and nervous tissue which stimulates smooth muscle and dilates blood vessels, prostaglandins (q.v.) and gamma-amino-butyric acid (GABA) which is present in the central nervous system where it appears to inhibit nervous activity, possibly as a modulator of intensity of response to a given stimulus rather than as a direct transmitter substance. Such activity may explain the efficacy as a tranquilliser of haloperidol which is chemically related to GABA (see also 'Meprobamate').

Histamine
Despite its wide action in the body, the therapeutic uses of this compound are limited. Attempts have been made to employ it specifically to desensitize patients who have been thought on somewhat empirical grounds to be suffering from diseases due to histamine, but these have not been generally successful. At the moment histamine is used mainly in diagnosis in a test designed to demonstrate the secretion of acid by the stomach, a process which is stimulated in part by the drug and is not opposed by anti-histamines. Acid secretion does not occur in response to histamine in anaemia due to defective absorption of vitamin B_{12} (see 'Vitamin'), or following division of the main nerve supply to the stomach (vagotomy); in the latter case the test is used to check on the completeness of this operation.

Hydrocortisone

(Synthesized: as one of a group of twenty-eight crystalline compounds between 1930 and 1943 by Reichstein and co-workers. Trade names, in various chemical forms: Efcortelan sodium, Efcortesol, Hydro-adreson, Hydrocortistab, Hydrocortisyl, Hydrocortisone, Solu-Cortef, Cortisol, Cortef, Cortifan, Cortril, Hycortole, Hydrocortone, Cortef fluid, Magnacort. Administration: oral, rectal and injection.

Classification

The main natural hormone produced by the adrenal gland (see 'Hormones'). Originally prepared as an extract of adrenal gland, and subsequently identified as one of a mixture of twenty-eight compounds in such extracts. Its synthesizers, Reichstein and Kendall, received a Nobel Prize in Medicine for this work in conjunction with Hench who showed the efficacy of the compound in rheumatoid arthritis. Since then 'manipulations of structure have yielded a bewildering variety of synthetic analogues, *a few of which* represent modest therapeutic gains. . . .'*

Some of these synthetic 'corticosteroids' are cortisone (also a natural product), prednisone, prednisolone, paramethasone, methyl-prednisolone, triamcinolone, betamethasone, dexamethasone, fludrocortisone, deoxycortone acetate and aldosterone (also produced naturally by the adrenal gland).

Therapeutic uses

Perhaps in part because of the variety of preparations available, the place of corticosteroids in the therapy of disease today is ill-defined. The different synthetic compounds vary in their anti-inflammatory potency in the treatment of such diseases as rheumatoid arthritis, asthma, conjunctivitis and ulcerative colitis, but such variations can be taken care of by alteration of dosage. With rare exceptions, the only real advantages from using one preparation rather than another is in the decrease of side effects, particularly of fluid retention, and of catabolism (see 'Metabolism'). The table on page 139 compares some of the more commonly used corticosteroids and gives an indication of their relative activities.

Perhaps the earliest use of corticosteroids was to replace the natural substance in patients with decreased adrenal activity, either acute due to sudden destruction of the adrenals, or chronic due to surgery or disease. In these cases it is usual to administer a steroid with potent salt-retaining ability. 9α-Fluoro-cortisol or aldosterone are usually used, the latter commonly with hydrocortisone. In another form of decreased adrenal function the

* Goodman and Gilman, *op. cit.*, p. 1609 (our italics).

Steroid	Relative anti-inflammatory effect	Relative salt-retaining effect	Relative catabolic effect
Hydrocortisone	1·0	1·0	—
Prednisone	3·5	0·8	4·8
Prednisolone	4·0	0·8	2·8
6α-Methyl-prednisolone	5·0	0·5	—
Triamcinolone	5·0	0·0	2·2
Paramethasone	10·0	0·0*	1·0
Betamethasone	25·0	0·0	2·4
Dexamethasone	25·0	0·0	1·4
9α-Fluoro-cortisol	15·0	125·0	—

— No figure available.
* Causes salt loss.

glands instead of being small or destroyed appear to be grossly enlarged, although definite symptoms of hormone deficiency may be present. In this condition, which is present at birth, the defect is biochemical, rather than physical, and the production of hydrocortisone is diminished. Thus the feedback inhibition of the pituitary is decreased, and in consequence it produces large quantities of ACTH causing the adrenal enlargement. Administered corticosteroid replaces that not being synthesized and also inhibits the abnormally increased production of excess adrenal androgens (see 'Testosterone') which give rise to virilizing side effects.

When administered to man or experimental animals, corticosteroids cause a decrease in the activity of the tissues which form the lymphocytes, one type of white blood cell. Thus they are effective in the treatment of leukaemia, particularly acute or chronic lymphocytic leukaemia. The steroids are often used in conjunction with anti-metabolites (see 'Actinomycin D', 'Methotrexate', '5-Fluorouracil', 'Chlorambucil').

Suppression of the lymphoid system (the tissues which produce lymphocytes), which also produces antibodies, is one of the prime aims of the use of corticosteroids in such diseases as Hodgkin's disease (see 'Azathioprine', 'Methotrexate') as well as in organ transplantation. Here the donor organ acts like any other foreign protein to the recipient body and stimulates antibody production to itself. By diminishing the activity of the lymphoid system, and also by inhibiting inflammatory reactions, corticosteroids prevent rejection and prolong the life of the transplanted organ. However, they also inhibit the body's defence against infection. It is for this reason that transplant patients must be nursed in special sterile facilities, where the attending doctor must continually walk the tight-rope of dosage between infection on the one hand and rejection on the other.

The activity of hydrocortisone and related synthetic compounds in diminishing immunity reactions is seen to the full in their use to treat acute asthmatic attacks. The narrowing of the air passages to the lungs is thought to be due to changes brought about by the release of histamine (see 'Aspirin', 'Tripelennamine', 'Hormone') as a result of a reaction on the surface of the cells lining these passages between a protein foreign to the body (antigen) and antibodies. Usually these changes occur in response to some substance such as pollen to which the sufferer is then said to be allergic. Although corticosteroids have not been shown to interfere with the antibody–antigen reaction and consequent histamine release, they inhibit the inflammatory response to cell damage which follows.

The effect of corticosteroids on immunity reactions may also explain their use in the treatment of rheumatoid arthritis, a degenerative disease in which the joints are gradually destroyed and eventually fuse (see 'Indomethacin'). The condition may be an auto-immune disease (see 'Azathioprine') in which the defences of the body that give immunity against foreign substances suddenly attack its own joint-lining tissues. Thus, suppression of the lymphoid tissue by these agents could control the degeneration. Another school of thought ascribes the joint changes to cell damage such as that which produces inflammation. Intracellular organelles called lysosomes which contain enzymes used to break down (lyse) unwanted molecules become more easily broken. The lytic enzymes are released and cellular damage results. The ability of corticosteroids to increase the resistance of the membrane which forms a lysosome and encloses the enzymes, so that it is less liable to break, could explain their efficacy in treatment (see 'Fluocinolone acetonide').

Other diseases in which the use of corticosteroids is advocated largely because the cause is thought to be due to development of resistance by the body to its own tissues (auto-immunity) include ulcerative colitis in which the steroid given through the rectum may bring dramatic relief, a kidney disease in which it has been alleged that up to two-thirds of children so affected may recover completely, and a severe and rapidly fatal disease, systemic lupus erythematosus, in which the blood vessels in the skin, joints and kidney (the last leading to death from renal failure) are affected. Acute episodes of this disease may be successfully treated with corticosteroids and allow the introduction of other less drastic forms of therapy.

Hydrocortisone can be applied to the skin for the treatment of skin disease (see 'Fluocinolone acetonide').

Side effects
Corticosteroids have been associated with practically every conceivable side effect, but many of them occur only after enormous doses over prolonged periods of time. Certainly distinct metabolic (see 'Metabolism') and associated changes can occur which are in general expressions of the normal physiological or pharmacological activities of the compounds, but by careful selection of specific synthetic compounds (because they vary in their effects), and by dosage at prescribed times of day, it is often possible to avoid these changes except in the most minimal form.

Steroids cause salt to be retained in the body. This is particularly the case with prednisone and prednisolone which still represent about sixty per cent of all steroid prescriptions (presumably because they are cheap). Because of the salt-retention, their use is frequently associated with local tissue fluid accumulation (see 'Diuretic'). This complication may be sufficiently severe to cause heart failure. Surprisingly, however, one of these preparations, paramethasone acetate, has actually been used in cases of heart failure; presumably because of its *salt-losing* capacity, it has been successful in promoting diuresis.

Redistribution of body fat, as well as water, is seen with corticosteroids and gives rise to the typical 'mooning' of the face and 'buffalo hump' due to accumulation of fat between the shoulder-blades.

Stimulation of glucose production by steroids causes an increase in blood-sugar, with the appearance of glucose in the urine. Thus a condition commonly called steroid diabetes (see 'Insulin') may be produced which responds to normal diabetic therapy. Gastric acid production is increased, too, and this may cause ulceration.

Corticosteroids are catabolic (see 'Metabolism') particularly in muscles and bone. In the former they may cause muscle weakness, notably around the shoulders and pelvis; in the latter they cause loss of calcium as a consequence of loss of bone structure, although these changes are usually only associated with long-term treatment. Thinning of the skin, and bruising due to weakness of blood vessels, are occasionally seen with corticosteroid treatment, and these also are catabolic effects.

The use of steroids to diminish inflammation also leads to side effects, particularly in the form of decreased resistance to infection. After their use, even minor infections such as a 'boil' can overwhelm the body's resistance. Vigorous antibiotic treatment is required under these circumstances.

The early use of large quantities of corticosteroids in children, for example, for leukaemia, caused considerable stunting of growth. This is now known to be due to an alteration of the cartilage, specialized growth tissue at the end of bones, and to decreased absorption of calcium from the gut, apparently by antagonizing the effects of vitamin D (see 'Vitamin'). Calcium is needed for bone formation.

Cortisol effects in the brain may cause psychosis. Both cortisol deficiency and excess cause alteration of the electrical activity of the brain, which cannot be due simply to altered electrolyte (q.v.) metabolism as it is not reversed by the administration of the salt-retaining steroid deoxycorticosterone. The other main side effect of the corticosteroids is adrenal suppression. In times of stress, for example, at operation, the adrenal responds by pouring out large quantities of cortisol. In patients who have been treated for periods of time with corticosteroids, however, this may not always occur. A few fatalities have occurred, allegedly due to prolonged corticosteroid treatment with irreversible adrenal suppression. Although opinion is divided about the significance of this effect, and the need to anticipate it, such patients are commonly helped over an operation with extra intravenous hydrocortisone.

Chemistry and physiology

The actions of the corticosteroids can be approximately divided into two: the carbohydrate (glucose) regulating activity (glucocorticoid action), which correlates with clinical anti-inflammatory action; and the electrolyte (salt and water) regulating activity (mineralocorticoid action). Different compounds vary in their relative activities.

The glucocorticoid activity of corticosteroids is considerable. It is generally agreed that this is partly due to increased release of protein and amino acids (see 'Biochemistry') from muscles, and it has been suggested that formation of new liver enzymes (q.v.) for conversion of amino acids to glycogen (a large carbohydrate molecule which is in effect the cellular store of smaller glucose molecules) is aided by the drugs.

Fat metabolism is also affected by corticosteroids, as indeed is almost every major metabolic function in the body. The mode of action is not yet clear, but preliminary evidence (1969) suggests that corticosteroids will increase the fat-mobilizing effect of adrenaline (q.v.), hours being required for effects. The increase is blocked by inhibitors of ribonucleic acid (RNA) or protein synthesis, suggesting that the metabolic change occurs because cells produce new enzymes, or more of those which they already synthesize.

The mineralocorticoids, particularly aldosterone, affect sodium, potassium and associated water metabolism. These compounds may act at the level of the distal tubule in the kidney (see 'Diuretic') and increase sodium reabsorption. Here again, as in the case of fat metabolism, cells may be synthesizing additional enzymes that are involved in sodium transport. The production of aldosterone is thought to be controlled by a compound, angiotensin II, whose production is itself controlled by renin from the juxta-glomerular apparatus (a specialized group of cells close to the filtration unit of the kidney which respond to lower blood pressure by increasing their output of renin). Thus low blood pressure due, for example, to blood loss and shock can lead to sodium and water retention to make up for the fluid lost.

The effects on the cardiovascular system are probably due mainly to those on the electrolyte (q.v.) levels which significantly affect heart contractility, although an effect on the capillaries is also possible. Corticosteroids have been implicated in the development of hypertension, but it is now thought that they play a 'permissive' role, allowing other factors to operate.

Abnormalities of muscle function can appear both in adrenal insufficiency and after administration of large doses of corticosteroids, a seemingly paradoxical situation. In the former this is due to diminished circulation to the muscle with consequent lack of essential nutrients while in the latter the effects can be attributed to the muscle-wasting activity of the steroids.

Theories advanced to explain the effects of the corticosteroids in the central nervous system ('Side effects', above) range from suggestions that cortisol acts by maintaining cerebral blood flow, to complex hypotheses involving multiple actions at different levels of the brain and indeed in different organs with secondary cerebral effects. Two of the more attractive theories involve an interaction between the circulating levels of corticosteroid and substances thought to act either as brain transmitters (that is, a chemical which serves to carry a nervous impulse from one nerve cell to another; see 'Adrenaline', 'Atropine'), or as modulators of brain-cell activity. It has been suggested that excess cortisol in the blood causes an increase in liver enzymes which lead to lowered levels of 5-hydroxytryptamine (5-HT), probably one of the brain transmitters, particularly in an area associated with the 'production' of depression (for further discussion see 'Imipramine'). Alternatively cortisol levels may change the level of gamma-amino-butyric acid (GABA) which is thought to act as an inhibitory modulator of transmission in the brain, raised cortisol levels diminishing brain GABA with consequent nervous excitation. While there is evidence for both theories, at present the physiological action of cortisol in causing nervous changes remains unclear.

The cellular mechanism of action of cortisol, as with other steroids, is also not completely clear. There is evidence that this type of compound can cause increase in availability of deoxyribonucleic acid (DNA) for RNA synthesis, and that it is bound specifically to nuclei where DNA and RNA are largely formed. However, much of this work has been done in the liver, which is a site of inactivation of cortisol rather than an organ which responds specifically to the hormone, and its significance is therefore uncertain. Other evidence suggests that corticosteroids act by altering the passage of substances across the membrane that encloses cells or the organelles within them ('Therapeutic uses', above). Such findings would accord with the opinions of those who ascribe the effects of the steroids to changes in electrolyte levels. It seems possible that a final common mode of action of corticosteroids at the cellular level will eventually be found; in view of the enormous differences which may be produced by minor molecular alterations, it is no doubt complex.

Imipramine

(Synthesized: Häfliger, 1948, Switz.) Trade names: Tofranil, Berkomine. Administration: oral, injection.

Classification
An anti-depressant drug closely related chemically to chlor-promazine (q.v.), one of a class called tricyclics because of their molecular structure. The only other tricyclic anti-depressant in regular use is amitryptiline (Laroxyl, Saroten, Triptafen, Tryptizol; U.S.: Elavil).

Therapeutic uses
Imipramine and amitryptiline have brought improvement in 60–70 per cent of depressed patients to whom the drugs have been given. This is a better record than that of the monoamine

oxidase (MAO) inhibitors (see 'Phenelzine'), the other major class of anti-depressant compounds. However, the tricyclics are most useful against endogenous depression whereas the MAO inhibitors are more valuable for reactive or neurotic depression.

Like many mental illnesses (and not a few somatic diseases), depression is a poorly defined condition ranging over a continuum from those sad days that seem to be part of the 'normal' human condition to the suicidal hopelessness of a psychotic. Broadly speaking, depressive illness is classified as endogenous when there seem to be no outward, objective causes such as disease, business failure, death of a loved one or some blow to the patient's self-esteem. These patients are often older. Reactive depression, on the other hand, is traceable to some external event, though the patient's reaction to it is considered by the doctor, the patient's family or the patient himself to be too extreme. Reactive depression is often associated with irregular periods of irrational fear, and severe phobic anxiety in which the patient is frightened of some place like an open field, or a thing like a snake.

Imipramine has also been useful for the treatment of enuresis (bed-wetting) in both children and adults.

Side effects

By and large, the tricyclic anti-depressants are safer than the MAO inhibitors. Like them, however, imipramine requires two to three weeks before it begins to affect the patient's mood, but side effects can occur much faster. About 10 per cent of those given imipramine develop a fine tremor, and older patients may suffer severe sudden tremors and Parkinson-like symptoms (see 'L-Dopa'). High doses can cause epileptic seizures. Acute overdosage manifests itself as fever, high blood pressure, seizures and coma. The convulsions can be controlled with short-acting barbiturates (see 'Phenobarbitone'), and high blood pressure with phenoxybenzamine (q.v.) or drugs with similar modes of action. Physical methods must be used to control fever. Heart irregularities are the most serious symptom of tricyclic poisoning, however, and can be the hardest to correct. Even with lower doses of these drugs chronic disturbances in heart rhythms may develop, and the blood pressure may fall when the patient stands erect.

Less serious side effects can include constipation, dizziness, palpitations, blurred vision, urine retention, excessive sweating, weakness, fatigue and headache. Amitryptiline may produce fewer of these side effects, but it is more sedative than imipramine. Older patients are more subject to all of these minor untoward reactions.

Continuance of the drug will often be accompanied with diminution in the less serious side effects due to the development of tolerance for the drug. Patients who have taken imipramine for many months may display mild withdrawal symptoms if the drug is removed, but there is no evidence that it is addictive.

Imipramine given with an MAO inhibitor can cause severe reactions. At least a week should separate the use of the two types of drugs.

Chemistry and physiology

The mechanism of action of the tricyclic anti-depressants is not known. Part of the difficulty arises out of the problem of defining depression. Unlike the common cold or measles, it is not a clearcut disease with objective causes and measurable symptoms. On the contrary, both the patient and the doctor are making their diagnosis on the basis of subjective judgements: the patient feels unhappy and the doctor thereupon identifies a treatable disease. Similarly, when a drug is given to the patient, his reaction is subjective; indeed, the only measurable indications that the drug is acting may be undesirable side effects such as disturbances in heart rhythm.

Since so many of the less serious side effects produced by imipramine are like those induced by atropine (q.v.), it has been suggested that the tricyclics affect the metabolism (q.v.) of acetylcholine (ACh), one of the chemical transmitters of nervous signals across gaps between neurons and from neurons to cells in muscles or glands. There is also some evidence, however, that these drugs increase the available amounts of another chemical transmitter, noradrenaline (see 'Adrenaline').

The question is, of course, what connexions exist between these biological chemicals and the disease called depression. The existing evidence is extremely limited. Depression may occur when the amount of noradrenaline falls below normal at neurons in a brain centre called the amygdala, for example. The amygdala may be the site of distinctive nerve clusters that regulate feelings of pleasure and anger or pain. Along with other nearby centres, the amygdala is almost certainly responsible for the regulation of emotional responses. Additional evidence implicates a third chemical transmitter of nervous messages, 5-hydroxytryptamine (5-HT), which is also believed to act between some nerve cells in the amygdala, and may be in abnormally short supply in depressed patients. In any case, noradrenaline can be shown to excite amygdaloid neurons, and 5-HT inhibits their activity. However, other substances such as dopamine (see 'L-Dopa') may also be transmitters between nerve cells in centres closely related to the amygdala, and dopamine metabolism may also be altered by antidepressant drugs. It seems probable that the symptoms of depression are related to imbalance among the natural transmitters of nervous messages between brain cells. It is possible that such biochemical imbalances are triggered by environmental conditions.

The symptoms of depression are related to those of anxiety on the one hand, and may blend into those of mania on the other. MAO inhibitors are thought to act on the metabolism of 5-HT. These antidepressants are useful not only in the control of reactive depression but also for anxiety (see 'Chlorpromazine', 'Tranquillizer'). The tricyclics, on the other hand, may exacerbate anxiety. It seems probable, therefore, that anxiety and depression share some biochemical as well as symptomatic similarities, but that the two conditions can also be differentiated biochemically. Despite the chemical relation between the molecule of chlorpromazine (q.v.) and that of imipramine, moreover, chlorpromazine is useful in the treatment of anxiety.

In some depressed patients, both the tricyclic and the MAO inhibitor drugs can cause episodes of excitement and mania. The fact that both classes of compounds can produce such effects is evidence for the hypothesis that mania is a reflection of biochemical changes similar to but more extreme than those that underlie depression. Mania and occasionally depression itself can also be controlled with lithium salts. Lithium is a natural metallic element like potassium, one of the positive ions (q.v.) normally found inside nerve cells. Lithium may be poisonous. It replaces potassium ions inside nerve cells, thus disrupting their functions, and it also alters characteristics of the membrane that surrounds nerve cells (as well as all other cells). Both the membrane and the movement of ions through it into and out of nerve cells play a role in their excitability, and lithium does alter excitability. It is possible that tricyclics and MAO inhibitors also alter the characteristics and behaviour of nerve cell membranes, and indeed, that the disease symptoms arise from malfunctions at the cell membrane. It may not be the amounts of the transmitter chemicals that are abnormal, but rather the way they act at the membranes.

At present, it is possible only to suggest that depression, mania, anxiety and other psychic disturbances reflect biophysical malfunctions involving transmitter chemicals and their receptors on cell membranes. The so-called neuroleptic drugs, those that appear to correct psychic disease symptoms, including the anti-depressants, act somehow in this context.

Indomethacin

(Sarrett, *et al.*, 1961, U.S.) Trade names: Indocid (U.K.), Indocin (U.S.). Administration: orally, in capsules or tablets, and in suppositories.

Classification

Synthesized in the course of a search for an anti-inflammatory drug which would produce the desirable effects of steroids (see 'Hormone') such as hydrocortisone (q.v.) without their unwanted side effects. Indomethacin is chemically related to an important natural substance, 5-hydroxytryptamine (5-HT, serotonin) which is thought to be a chemical messenger bearing impulses between juxtaposed nerve ends in parts of the brain, and possibly in other tissues as well (see 'Phenelzine'). Research leading to discovery of the agent began with the hypothesis that 5-HT played a role in the inflammatory process, a view that has since been abandoned.

Therapeutic uses

The drug has pain-killing (analgesic) and fever-reducing (antipyretic) properties as well as anti-inflammatory effects. It is used to treat the symptoms of rheumatic and arthritic disorders, notably osteo-arthritis, rheumatoid arthritis and spinal arthritis (ankylosing spondylitis). It is also administered in combination with a uricosuric (see 'Allopurinol') such as phenylbutazone to treat gout, but indomethacin is the drug of choice for relief from acute gouty attacks because of its speed of action. In the treatment of arthritis, the agent may require two to four months to achieve its maximum therapeutic effect.

Side effects

These may include dizziness, headache, loss of appetite, nausea, vomiting, diarrhoea and gastrointestinal disorders, the most serious of which is peptic ulcers. Indomethacin should not be given to patients who have or have had peptic ulcers. Drowsiness, confusion, blurred vision, faintness, psychotic disturbances, rash and excess body fluid (oedema) occur less frequently. Some blood disturbances have also been reported in patients with rheumatoid arthritis. All of these side effects appear to be reversible when the drug is withdrawn. Headache, a fairly common effect, may be controlled by the simultaneous administration of an antihistamine (see 'Tripelennamine').

Chemistry and physiology

Indomethacin is an indole derivative, as is 5-HT. Its mechanism of action is unknown.

The drug appears to control inflammation directly; that is, at the swollen joints. Like aspirin (q.v.), it probably reduces inflammation and the related pain and fever by blocking biosynthesis of prostaglandins (q.v.).

Rheumatic diseases are inflammatory conditions of the musculoskeletal system. When the body joints themselves are involved, the condition is called arthritis. If connective tissue near joints or around muscle and tendon suffers, the disease may be called fibrositis. Bursitis is inflammation of sac-like spaces (bursa) filled with fluid at positions where they can reduce friction. Gout is a form of joint disease in which the cause of inflammation is thought to be crystals composed of uric acid which precipitate out of body fluids at the site (see 'Allopurinol'). This closely related group of disorders causes more physical suffering and economic loss than perhaps any other disease state. They have been recognized, furthermore, at least since 8000 B.C. according to Egyptian records. Yet their cause or causes are largely unknown, and their classification and diagnosis erratic and uncertain.

All moving joints in the body are composed of bone and cartilage (a tough, tendinous substance unlike bone in formation and structure), lined with a soft, smooth, cellular substance called the synovial lining. These cells secrete a substance called synovial fluid into the space or capsule enclosed by the lining. The fluid lubricates the joint. In arthritis, various distortions of these arrangements may occur: the synovial cells can cease secreting fluid so that the joint 'dries out'; the cells can alter the chemical character and therefore the physical properties of the fluid, or they can die so that the joint becomes semirigid like bone.

In 1969 a virus was for the first time implicated in such changes. Although they are clearly metabolic in nature, and may involve cellular overproduction of hydrogen ions (q.v.), the exact biochemical differences between normal and abnormal cells is unclear. The chemical composition of normal synovial fluid is of course known, and it can be synthesized and even injected into arthritic joints, but with practically no lasting effect. It is thought that at least certain forms of rheumatism, particularly those associated with rheumatoid arthritis, may be auto-immune diseases; i.e., malfunctions which arise when cells which normally produce antibodies against substances foreign to the body begin instead to manufacture antibodies which attack the body's own cells. Such a shift in cell metabolism would possibly require a mutation in the genetic material of the cell, but why or how this happens remains a subject for research and speculation.

Early in 1969, it was announced that special forms of vitamin C and K (q.v.) may correct the metabolic disturbances of the synovial cells. For the present, however, the treatment of rheumatic disorders, with the possible exception of gout, remains symptomatic: drugs reduce the inflammation, and therefore, the pain and swelling. Indomethacin, phenylbutazone, hydrocortisone (q.v.) and aspirin (q.v.), each in their own way, are among the agents which have proved useful.

Insulin

(Extracted: Banting and Best, 1921–2, Canada; structure established: Sanger, 1960, U.S.; synthesized: Katsoyannis, 1964). Trade names: none ('Classification', below). Administration: injection.

Classification
A natural hormone (q.v.) formed in tissue segments of the pancreas called Islets of Langerhans (see description of pancreas under 'Hormone'). Most of the preparations used clinically are extracts from the pancreas of cattle or hogs. However, the drug may be modified synthetically to give it longer-acting qualities. Whereas pure insulin acts for about six hours, isophane insulin suspension (isophane insulin) and insulin zinc suspension (lente insulin) have a duration of about twenty-four hours, and protamine zinc insulin suspension and extended zinc insulin suspension (ultra-lente insulin), about thirty-six hours. Duration varies with the dose and the individual patient. Mixtures of some of these preparations may be used.

Therapeutic uses
With dietary control, regulation of weight and exercise, and possibly oral anti-diabetic drugs (see 'Chlorpropamide'), insulin is used for the control of diabetes mellitus, a disease characterized in the first instance by abnormally high glucose (see 'Biochemistry') content of the blood and urine. The metabolic disturbances related to the disease affect not only the use of sugar, however, but also of protein and fat. So interrelated are these substances in terms of their chemical structures as well as their roles in living organisms that the aberrant metabolism (q.v.)

of diabetes is enormously complex. Treatment is inevitably both subtle and multi-faceted, though insulin can always be useful if its administration is most carefully regulated.

Two forms of the disease are recognized: early-onset diabetes occurs before the age of twenty, is often accompanied by weight loss and apathy, and stems from partial or complete failure of insulin production. Late-onset diabetes occurs after the age of forty and not before thirty; the patient usually suffers from obesity, and the condition appears to be unrelated to pancreatic production of insulin, which may indeed be greater than normal. Early-onset diabetes customarily responds well to insulin therapy, but the late-onset variety may be better controlled by rigid diet regulation, exercise and oral drugs. In acute diabetic conditions related to the late-onset form, however, massive doses of insulin are required to save life.

One such acute condition, which can arise in both forms of the disease, is called diabetic ketoacidosis, or ketosis. It can lead to respiratory disorders, insufficiencies of essential electrolytes (q.v.) such as sodium and potassium, and cumulative central nervous disruption culminating in diabetic coma and death.

Although the disease is always accompanied by an insufficiency of insulin, whether absolute or relative to the availability of the hormone in active form, its causes are unknown. Several factors have been implicated in its development. Malformed antibodies (see 'Azathioprine') or other protein molecules in the blood and tissue fluid (lymph) of diabetics, but not of normal persons, bind chemically to insulin molecules so that the latter are inactivated, perhaps because they are structurally distorted by the chemical linkage.

Cortisol (see 'Hydrocortisone') and two additional hormones (q.v.) – adrenocorticotrophic hormone (ACTH) and growth hormone (GH) – normally have metabolic effects opposite to those of insulin. ACTH regulates the secretion of cortisol by the adrenal cortex, and cortisol increases the amount of glucose in the body by mediating biosynthesis of the sugar, chiefly in the liver, from stores of fat and from protein. GH plays a role in normal growth, as the name suggests; the substance also both increases glucose supply from fat and protein, and inhibits its use by muscle and liver cells.

Factors may exist, furthermore, which compete with insulin molecules for target sites within cells so that the hormone cannot function properly when it is present. There is some evidence, principally of a statistical nature, that some or all of these developmental phenomena stem from mutations in cells of lymph- and blood-forming tissue so that diabetes is an auto-immune disease (see 'Azathioprine').

Side effects

Untoward reactions to insulin can include itching or pain at the site of injection, and allergic reactions to the animal hormone, which may be extreme. The most serious side effect, however, is insulin shock caused by overdosage. Insulin shock may first manifest itself in hunger, nausea, gastrointestinal discomfort, slowed heartbeat, lethargy and impairment of brain functions. These symptoms are followed by rapid breathing, sweating and increased blood pressure and heart rate. In its later stages, insulin shock, like diabetic ketosis, produces convulsions, coma and permanent brain damage or death. Though caused by directly antagonistic events, in the late stages these two conditions are clinically similar. In insulin shock there is too little blood sugar so that glucose must be given and insulin treatment temporarily stopped. In ketoacidosis there is too much blood sugar so that insulin therapy must be intensive.

Chemistry and physiology

Insulin cannot be given orally because it is a protein and would be denatured in the digestive tract. The mechanisms by which it acts in the body, physiologically or pharmacologically, are unclear. The protein contains fifty-one amino acid bases in two chains linked together by sulphur bound to hydrogen (sulphydryl bonds). The exact conformation of the molecule has been described, so that it should soon be possible to identify its active sites. Once these are known, it may become possible to locate the target molecules in or on body cells.

Three theories of action have been advanced, for all of which there is some experimental evidence. Indeed, the theories are supportive rather than exclusive. It was first proposed that insulin altered the molecular structure of cell membranes so that they would admit hexoses, a class of six-carbon sugars which includes glucose, to the cell. Without insulin, the intracellular machinery grinds to a halt because the requisite fuel is not available. Thus, according to this hypothesis, diabetes reflects starvation in the midst of plenty.

A second theory implicates insulin in the normal formation of glycogen, the glucose polysaccharide in which form sugar is stored in animals, principally by liver and muscle cells. Insulin has been shown to have a stimulating effect on the biosynthesis of glycogen such that without the hormone, free glucose remains unutilized within cells (where it cannot all be used up at the same time), and therefore in the extracellular fluids as well.

The failure of glucose to enter cells and the absence of stored glycogen trigger the body to search for other, non-carbohydrate sources of energy. Fat stores and protein are brought from various tissues to the liver, the major storage site for glycogen, where they are broken down, but instead of being synthesized into glucose or glycogen, they are formed into ketone bodies. Ketones are chemicals which contain a keto group (CO); there are three biological ketone bodies: acetone (CH_3COCH_3), aceto-acetic acid (CH_3COCH_2COOH) and beta-hydroxybutyric acid ($CH_3CH(OH)CH_2COOH$). Overproduction of these substances disrupts the sensitive acid-base balance maintained in health by adding excess acids to body fluids. This is the condition known as diabetic ketosis. Yet evidence indicates that at least in normal individuals ketones may also encourage the secretion of insulin.

It would at first appear that disturbances in protein and fat metabolism are caused by the malfunctions in carbohydrate (particularly sugar) metabolism. Once again, however, the biosynthetic processes are more complex: there is evidence that insulin exerts a direct effect at least on protein biosynthesis, and that without the hormone, amino acids are less efficiently incorporated into protein. Thus, the third theory of insulin action holds that it is in some degree instrumental in the normal formation of protein.

The object of diabetic therapy is to reduce the sugar levels in blood and urine, and to prevent the build-up of ketones. Insulin normally promotes these objectives, but the same factors which can contribute to development of the disease may cause a 'resistance' to the therapy. Apparent insulin resistance due to blood-protein binding of the hormone, the antagonistic action of adrenal or pituitary hormones or other factors is just as much a 'cause' of diabetes as is insulin lack. In treatment, however, insulin resistance must often be overcome by doses so large that they could be fatal to the patient who lacks insulin entirely and is, therefore, more sensitive to it. Diagnostic distinctions between the early- and late-onset forms of the disease and among the metabolic disturbances which can occur at any time in the course of it are essential.

Interferon

(Isaacs and Lindemann, 1957, U.K.) The compound is not used in clinical practice.

Interferon is a small protein molecule formed in the cells of man and other mammals when they are invaded by viruses and certain bacteria-like organisms. It is not an official drug because it has not been purified or described chemically, nor has injection of interferon-containing extracts prevented disease in experimental animals. Nevertheless, the discovery of the substance has enormous importance in the recent history of pharmacology: its existence seemed to prove that cells possess a natural defence against viral infections. If interferon could be got into the cells, or if cells could be induced to synthesize or release more of the substance, or if its mechanism of anti-viral action could be mimicked by other agents, drugs specific against flu, smallpox, polio and the hundreds of other diseases caused by viruses might be found.

In fact, this expectation has been partially fulfilled. Some six synthetic anti-viral drugs now exist. Amantadine (trade name: Symmetrel) can prevent certain forms of influenza (the A_2 strains) if it is given before or at the time infection occurs, although evidence of resistant A_2 virus strains has been reported. The agent appears to alter the characteristics of cell membranes so that the virus particles cannot enter the cell to infect it (see below).

Methisazone (trade name: Marboran) prevents smallpox, but it too must be given before or at the time infection takes place. This compound works inside the cell to prevent the multiplication of viruses, in a manner which is thought to be analogous to interferon.

Idoxuridine (trade names: Dendrid, Stoxil, Herplex, Kerecid, U.S.) is probably the most widely used anti-viral drug, especially against certain viral infections of the eye, forms of encephalitis and skin disorders. It too works within the cell by disrupting the formation of new viral genetic material (deoxyribonucleic acid, DNA; see below), but it also distorts cellular DNA. Thus, it can have severe side effects such as damage to blood-cell-forming tissue and the mucosal lining of the intestinal tract.

Isoquinoline, a compound which has had some experimental success against B-type influenza infections in man, probably works by preventing intracellular viral replication (that is, the production of new viruses). Certain intestinal diseases have been controlled in animal studies by compounds called benzimidazoles, which are related to vitamin B_{12} (see 'Vitamin').

An antibiotic (q.v.), rifampicin, has also been found to prevent the multiplication of smallpox and related viruses as well as certain bacteria. Its action appears to prevent the synthesis of new viral (and bacterial) genetic material – in this case, ribonucleic acid (RNA). Although the agent has been used successfully against tuberculosis (see 'Isoniazid'), it has not been marketed as an anti-viral drug.

The most common anti-viral drugs are of course vaccines, which can prevent polio, measles, yellow fever and, more recently, rubella and mumps. The vaccines work because they stimulate the appropriate body cells to produce antibodies against the specific viral antigens (see discussion of immune responses under 'Azathioprine'). The antibodies destroy the virus before it can enter cells and multiply. Vaccination can also be used for the same purpose against bacteria; e.g. those causing diphtheria. But many of the most serious diseases caused by bacteria can now be cured after the infection begins by the use of antibiotics (q.v.) or sulphonamides (q.v.). These drugs either kill the bacteria or prevent their multiplication. Neither interferon, nor the other anti-viral drugs, stimulate the body's immune defences (except in so far as interferon is one of those defences), nor do they cure the infection by destroying the causative agent directly. Interferon is principally a prophylactic, i.e., it prevents the infection from occurring (below).

Chemistry and physiology

To explain the action of interferon (and of synthetic agents which have similar effects), it is necessary to describe the peculiar life-cycle of the organisms known collectively as viruses. With variations, a virus is in structure a molecule of genetic material, either DNA or RNA, surrounded by a tough coat consisting of one or more kinds of protein molecule, possibly linked with molecules of fat and, in some cases, of more RNA. Although they possess the genes which dictate the inheritance of characteristics by the next generation of viruses, these organisms lack the machinery, especially the intracellular organelles called ribosomes, by means of which all cells synthesize proteins, both enzymes (q.v.) and structural proteins. It is the proteins synthesized by the cell which allow it to express its functions, to grow and reproduce itself. In order for a virus to reproduce, however, it must get inside a cell where it can expropriate the available ribosomal machinery of the cell.

By means of certain molecules in their coat proteins, viruses attach themselves to the membranes of target cells. They then extrude their DNA or RNA core through the cell membrane into the cell. The old virus is now an inert protein coat, to all intents and purposes dead, whereas the cell is infected by the viral genetic material. Thus freed, the viral genes synthesize molecules within the cell which act as messengers between the genes and the cellular ribosomes, to 'instruct' the latter in manufacture of viral proteins. This viral messenger-RNA (m-RNA) displaces the m-RNA native to the cell at the ribosomes which then begin to produce proteins characteristic of the virus rather than of the cell. Eventually, new viral genetic material surrounded by new viral coats appear within the cell. These virions are released, usually by the destruction of the cell, and, as full grown viruses, can go on to locate and infect other cells. Thus, unlike cells, which only double their number from one generation to the next, viruses can reproduce themselves in multiples which are almost literally astronomical.

Although it is not directly relevant to the action of interferon, viruses may also behave in quite different ways when they infect a cell. Instead of at once expropriating the cellular ribosomes, the viral genetic material can combine with the cell's chromosomes. In this condition, the viral genes can remain latent for an indefinite period, behaving rather like recessive genes that already exist on the chromosome. Or the viral genes can express themselves along with the cellular genes in a manner which distorts the behaviour of the cell, but neither kills it nor causes it to produce new virions – at least not immediately. It may be that this latter viral behaviour is the cause of some forms of cancer.

To return to the infectious reproduction of viruses, however, certain aspects of the therapy of viral disease can now be explained. For example, the viral antigens which stimulate competent body cells to produce antibodies against them are probably one or more of the types of protein molecule which make up the tough viral coat. But the clearest understanding of the difficulties inherent in the chemotherapy of virus-caused diseases comes from a comparison of their life-cycles with that of bacteria. The latter are living cells which multiply outside body cells, utilizing their own manufacturing plant, so to speak. By determining metabolic differences between bacteria and body cells (and there are far more similarities than differences, in fact), it is possible to develop drugs which destroy the former while leaving the latter in relative peace. Viruses, on the other hand, multiply only by combining with body-cell machinery, so that compounds which prevent their multiplication are all too likely to be equally damaging to the cell. Because viruses multiply so rapidly within cells, furthermore, viral infection must be fully developed by the time disease symptoms appear. Bacterial infections develop more slowly; not only can drugs be used to stop their multiplication well before they have achieved a level of maximum growth – or infection – but also the body's natural defences have more time in which to mobilize against them.

Viruses have one more peculiarity which severely impedes the development of drugs against them. They are almost all highly species-specific; that is, a virus which causes flu in man, for example, will not infect monkeys or guinea pigs. Thus, it is not easy to test new drugs on living animals. Conversely, the drugs so far available are highly virus-specific; they control or prevent infection by a very limited number of viruses.

Interferon appears to be the major exception to this virus-specificity, which helps to explain its great importance. However, even this substance is species-specific. The interferon synthesized by human cells seems to differ in important ways from that produced by the cells of other mammals.

The action of interferon is by no means certain, but the compound is thought to alter the shape of the ribosomes so that the viral genetic material cannot bind to them while the cellular m-RNA remains free to do so.

Because interferon cannot yet be effectively administered as a drug, the attempt has been made to induce cells either to produce more of the substance or to release stores of it which are thought to be maintained within intracellular organelles. The first such inducer to be tried was a chemical called statolon. More recently, success has been achieved both in experimental animals and in man with a species of RNA which is double-stranded; that is, two complementary molecules of RNA are attached to each other in a double helix like that normally found in DNA. Why double-stranded RNA increases the amount of interferon in the cell is again unknown. However, double-stranded RNA has been shown to have toxic side effects so that there is renewed interest in the isolation and purification of interferon itself. A new agent, tilorone hydrochloride, has also been thought to cause the synthesis of interferon, at least in mice. Two compounds, one derived from starch and the other a synthetic called DEAE-fluoronone, may prove useful as interferon stimulators in man.

Ion

An atom with more or less than its normal complement of electrons, so that instead of being electrically neutral (that is, with the same number of electrons and protons – see 'Biochemistry'), it is either positively charged (because it lacks one or more electrons) or negatively charged. See also 'Electrolyte'.

Isoniazid

(Synthesized: Hoffmann La Roche Inc. and Squibb Institute for Medical Research, U.S., and Bayer, Ger., 1912; clinical use: Fox, 1952, U.S.) Trade names: Mybasan, Neumandin, Nicetal, Pycazide, Rimifon; also, containing aminosalicylate (see below): Carbopas, Dicosan, Inapasade, Minahpas, Nisapas, Nisogen, Pasinah, Pycamisan, Pycasix. Administration: oral, in tablets or syrup; injection.

Classification

A derivative of the vitamin (q.v.), nicotinamide (niacin). In 1945, it was accidentally found that the vitamin was useful in the treatment of tuberculosis. Other lines of research have been pursued in the development of drugs against this disease, but until the discovery of rifampicin, a new antibiotic (q.v.), none has been more successful.

Therapeutic uses

According to one authority, isoniazid is 'the keystone of the modern treatment of tuberculosis'.* The agent is used principally for treatment of tuberculosis of the lungs, but it is also effective against other forms of the disease, including tubercular meningitis and tuberculosis of the genito-urinary tract.

Isoniazid is frequently given with one or two other drugs, streptomycin (q.v.) and para-aminosalicylate, both to increase its effectiveness and to delay the emergence of resistance to the drug by the causative bacteria, *Mycobacteria tuberculosis.*

Side effects

These are related to dose and, with normal therapy, they are extremely rare. In most patients, those which occur will disappear when the drug is withdrawn. However, side effects can be severe and even fatal. Among the less frequent are dry mouth, loss of appetite, gastric upset, jaundice, pellagra and various blood disorders including anaemia. This form of anaemia is similar to one associated with a deficiency of pyridoxine (see 'Vitamin'), and it is thought that pyridoxine deficiency may also be the root cause of the peripheral neuritis which often accompanies higher-dose isoniazid therapy. The drug may in-

* A. Albert, *Selective Toxicity and Related Topics*, London, 1968, p. 343.

hibit the action of an enzyme (q.v.) which normally converts this vitamin into a substance which acts as a coenzyme in various processes of cellular energy conversion. Both the anaemia and the neuritis can often be prevented by simultaneous administration of vitamin B_6. Because it can alter the metabolism (q.v.) of isoniazid by cells, para-aminosalicylate may also diminish the occurrence of neuritis.

In patients with a history of epilepsy, high doses of isoniazid can bring on convulsions and must, therefore, be given to epileptics only with great care. Other central nervous effects can include muscle twitch, dizziness, ataxia, stupor, euphoria, psychoses and loss of memory. Optic neuritis may also occur. Rarely, isoniazid produces allergy-like reactions including fever, skin eruptions and hepatitis. The drug should not be given to people with certain kinds of kidney disease.

Chemistry and physiology

Isoniazid is bacteriostatic and may be bactericidal in man; that is, it halts the multiplication of the bacteria so that the body's normal defences can be mobilized to destroy them (and may actually kill them, also).

Its therapeutic action is thought to arise from effects which have no direct connexion with the pyridoxine competition which may cause the most serious side effects. *Mycobacteria tuberculosis* might be able to alter the drug metabolically so that it is built into nicotinamide adenine dinucleotide (NAD: see Niacin, under 'Vitamin') in place of nicotinamide. NAD is required for the process of energy conversion in cells, so that distortion of the molecule will cause the bacterium to stop growing, and eventually to die.

Isoniazid has revolutionized the treatment of tuberculosis, practically eliminating the need for sanatoria, and allowing a high percentage of cures. However, bacteria develop resistance to the compound whereupon it loses its therapeutic value. It has been estimated that about forty per cent of all *Mycobacteria tuberculosis* are normally resistant, probably because they are capable of synthesizing more of an enzyme (q.v.) which destroys the isoniazid molecule than can the non-resistant strains. As the non-resistant organisms are eliminated, therefore, the possibility exists that the resistant bacteria will grow in their place. Fortunately, there is no cross-resistance between isoniazid and streptomycin, para-aminosalicylate or other anti-tuberculosis drugs, though resistance to these agents also develops in time.

L-Dopa

(Experimental use: Cotzias, *et al.*, 1967, U.S.). Administration: oral.

Classification

A natural body substance, one of the precursors of noradrenaline, the chemical transmitter of nervous impulses between certain juxtaposed nerve ends and between some nerve ends and the muscles they control. L-Dopa is also a natural precursor of adrenaline (q.v.). Experiments with dopa were undertaken when it was discovered that the brain cells of patients suffering from Parkinson's disease contained less than the normal amount of dopamine, the intermediary chemical step in the biosynthesis of noradrenaline from dopa. It was reasoned that the subnormal supply of dopamine might cause the symptoms of the disease, but it was known that dopamine could not enter the brain from the bloodstream because of the membrane-like barrier which separates the brain from blood vessels. However, dopa – the immediate biological precursor of dopamine – does cross this blood-brain barrier, and it was, therefore, investigated.

Normally dopa consists of two different sets of molecules, each of which is a mirror image of the other. In crystalline form, these molecules can be distinguished from one another by the direction in which they bend a ray of polarized light. Those which bend the beam to the right are designated D (dextrorotatory) molecules, and their opposites, L (levo-rotatory). The roughly equal (racemic) natural mixture was relatively easy to obtain and purify, but it was found to cause a blood disorder in about a quarter of the patients who were given it. The pure L-form, on the other hand, does not have this side effect ('Side effects', below), but is much harder to purify and stabilize and, therefore, much more expensive.

Therapeutic uses

The only present use of L-Dopa is in the treatment of the symptoms of parkinsonism. The agent is the first important development in drug therapy for the disease in a century ('Chemistry and physiology', below). It is particularly helpful in restoration of control over voluntary movement, and for reduction or prevention of the crisis in which patients lose control of their eye muscles so that the eyeball moves erratically. The drug does not appear to prevent tremor in man. Indeed, clinical trials so far suggest that the compound helps only about half of those given it, although such a result is encouraging in the case of this disease.

It has been shown that high blood pressure in rats can be reduced by feeding L-Dopa. Whether this result will be found also in man remains to be demonstrated.

Side effects

With any new drug, side effects are still uncertain quantities, in part because correct dosage standards may not yet have been established. Thus, involuntary grimacing caused by L-Dopa can be stopped by reducing the dose, or slowing the rate at which it is being increased over a period of days. Restlessness, aggressiveness and delusions may be signs that the drug must be withdrawn altogether. Gastrointestinal effects are fairly frequent if the dosage is substantial. Nausea, and a fall in blood pressure, especially on standing erect, should disappear if dosage is held steady. Headache, sweating, panting and postural tremor are less frequent and will disappear if dose is reduced. The blood disorder caused by racemic D-, L-Dopa ('Classification', above) has also been reported with L-Dopa in two cases, and three cases of increased blood pressure are known. All unwanted reactions so far reported disappear when treatment with the drug is stopped, and no fatalities can be attributed to the compound. There has been a report that the drug has aphrodisiac qualities, but this could occur because of improvement in the patient's feelings of well being.

Perhaps the most serious side effect has emerged only from continued use, however. Tolerance to L-Dopa develops in most patients so that they require increasingly large doses to maintain the same improvement. Eventually, many patients develop symptoms such as extreme excitement of an almost manic quality, and themselves request the discontinuation of the drug. So far, it has been impossible to correct this situation once it arises.

Chemistry and physiology

At least three types of Parkinson's disease have been described. The causes are unknown, but there is evidence that decreased biosynthesis of dopamine due to a lack of the necessary enzyme (q.v.), L-aromatic amino acid decarboxylase, is a factor in the disorder.

The enzyme occurs in cells throughout the body, however, and may be indirectly responsible for the cardiovascular side effects of L-Dopa. Because decarboxylase functions in peripheral tissues, it converts some of the L-Dopa to dopamine outside the brain. Attempts are being made to control this reaction, and, incidentally, to reduce the required dose of an expensive drug, by adding decarboxylase inhibitors to the preparations. L-Dopa, like dopamine, noradrenaline and adrenaline, is a catecholamine (see 'Adrenaline'):

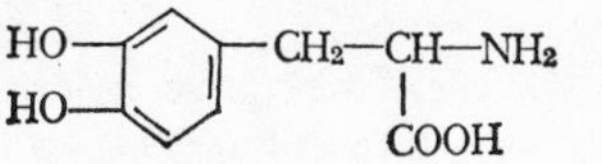

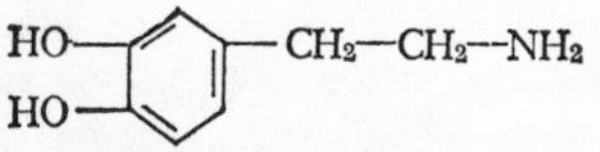

The most important earlier agents for treatment of parkinsonism are natural belladonna alkaloids, especially scopolamine (see 'Atropine'), and synthetic compounds chemically similar to them. L-Dopa differs from them both in structure and in mechanism of action.

Mepacrine. U.S.: Quinacrine

(Kikuth, 1930, Ger.) Also: atebrin. Trade name: Sobiacrin (contains mepacrine, chloroquine and other compounds). Administration: oral, or by intramuscular injection.

Classification
Synthesized during an intensive research programme in Germany instigated by the loss of quinine supplies during World War I. Chloroquine, primaquine and chlorguanide were developed by British and American research when Allied sources of quinine were lost during World War II, and have now largely replaced mepacrine in the treatment of malaria. Newer antimalarials include pyrimethamine. Quinine is rarely used clinically in developed countries today, except to combat organisms which cannot be destroyed by the synthetic drugs.

Therapeutic uses
Malaria continues to kill more people than any other disease, largely because it is endemic in the heavily populated, economic-

ally backward, warm regions. The disease is caused by one of four species of the *Plasmodium* family: *P. falciparum*, less frequent but often acute and fatal; *P. vivax*, perhaps the most common causative agent with a lower mortality and a high incidence of recurrence; *P. malariae* and *P. ovale*, both of which are relatively rare and less severe.

All parasites follow a similar life-cycle. Symptomatically inactive sporozoites are carried by mosquitoes, particularly the *Anopheles*, and injected into vertebrates by the insects. Sporozoites mature in body tissues, particularly in the liver, and appear in the blood as new organisms, merozoites, which enter red blood cells and multiply. Excepting for *P. falciparum*, however, some of these merozoites reinfect tissue cells where they are again symptomatically dormant. Eventually the red cells burst, releasing the parasites which can then infect other red cells. Some of the organisms released from red blood cells are unable to reproduce asexually; these gametocytes require the environment afforded by the mosquito's gut in order to reproduce new spores sexually. It is the destruction of red blood cells which causes the chills associated with the clinically active stage of the disease, and the foreign substances in the blood cause the fever as the result of an allergy-like reaction.

It would be most desirable to kill the spores before they can produce vegetative organisms, but no existing drugs will do this unless the dose level is poisonously high. Mepacrine and the other anti-malarials destroy the merozoites in the blood. Because *P. falciparum* does not reinfect tissues, cure of the disease is possible with existing agents when this organism is the cause. Vivax malaria has been cured by primaquine usually employed with chloroquine, but because of the reinfection of tissues by this organism, recurrence is frequent.

Like bacteria (see 'Antibiotic'), the malarial parasites develop resistance to drugs. This may be due to the prior existence of resistant strains as well as to mutations. In both cases, drugs tend to kill off the sensitive parasites, allowing the resistant organisms to flourish. Although resistance to one drug tends to extend to all of the anti-malarials, the organisms display less resistance to mepacrine, and are generally sensitive to quinine. Resistance also develops to the sulphonamides (q.v.), which have recently been pressed into service as anti-malarials, though evidence suggests that mepacrine may prevent the emergence of sulphonamide-resistant parasites, at least in some species of *Plasmodia*. So serious has this problem become from the clinical standpoint, however, that intensive efforts are now being directed once again to the destruction of the mosquito carriers, first by DDT, and with the discovery of the potential dangers inherent in that compound, by benzene hexachloride (BHC).

Mepacrine is also a drug of first choice to combat tapeworms and certain other species of worms. The agent has been used effectively against an unpleasant skin disease called lupus erythematosus.

Side effects

A huge number of soldiers were treated with mepacrine during World War II with a very low incidence of untoward reactions. Perhaps the most frequent is the slightly jaundiced cast the drug may give to the skin. It also can produce a rather pretty luminescent effect under nails and hair exposed to ultra-violet light.

Nausea, vomiting, abdominal cramps, headache, diarrhoea, vertigo, excessive sweating, fever, itching, insomnia and pains in muscles and joints may also be caused by the drug. All of these side effects disappear when treatment is stopped, but in a few cases, serious mepacrine poisoning affects the skin, the gastro-intestinal tract and central nervous system. It is these unusual toxic effects which have contributed to the displacement of mepacrine by chloroquine and primaquine, unless the organisms are resistant to these preferred drugs.

It has recently been suggested that the toxic effects can occur only in genetically predisposed individuals. For example, many Africans and natives of the Middle East are known to be deficient in an essential enzyme, glucose-6-phosphate dehydrogenase. Only patients with this inherited abnormality have developed a form of anaemia after treatment with primaquine.

Because they may affect the foetus, all of the anti-malarials should be administered to pregnant women only with the greatest caution.

Chemistry and physiology

The molecular mechanism of action of the anti-malarials is unclear, but they are now all thought to be anti-metabolites (see 'Metabolism',

'Chlorambucil', 'Methotrexate'); that is, compounds which inhibit some essential intracellular process. Mepacrine may kill *Plasmodia* because the drug molecule becomes inserted or intercalated into the deoxyribonucleic acid (DNA) of the cell. Correct replication of the gene-bearing molecule would thus be impeded, and the daughter cells would eventually die. Why this toxic effect is selective for the parasites and does not affect host cells is unknown.

Metabolism

'The sum of all the physical and chemical processes by which living organized substance is produced and maintained, and also the transformation by which energy is made available for the uses of the organism.'* Thus, cell metabolism, lymphocyte metabolism (see under 'Azathioprine'), bacterial metabolism, viral metabolism, human metabolism, etc., indicate that the processes are carried out in and by the specified organism; but drug metabolism refers to the uses which are made of the drug by living organisms, and also to the physical and chemical processes by which the drug is absorbed, altered and excreted by living organisms.

Anabolism is the sum of physical and chemical processes by which living organisms build up or construct substances which are in health necessary for their maintenance. However, the word is commonly used to describe the build-up or construction by living organisms of gross structures such as muscles. Biosynthesis commonly conveys the broader meaning of constructive metabolism. Catabolism refers to the breakdown or destruction of substances by living organisms. Thus, in common scientific usage biosynthesis and catabolism are opposites, whereas anabolism describes a more restricted group of events.

Metabolic is the adjectival form of metabolism. A metabolic activity is any process carried out by a living organism. It may be a biosynthetic or a catabolic process.

Metabolite is a substance used or produced by metabolism. Thus, glucose is a metabolite used for the production of energy (among other things); it is also a metabolite produced by the breakdown (catabolism) of glycogen (see 'Biochemistry').

Basal metabolism is the minimal energy expended by the body at rest to maintain its essential functions; e.g. respiration,

*Dorland's *Illustrated Medical Dictionary*, Philadelphia and London, 1965.

circulation, body temperature, etc. It is measured in units of heat; i.e. calories per square metre of body surface.

Methimazole

(Wohl and Marckwald, 1889, Ger.) Trade name: Tapazole. Administration: oral.

Classification

Methimazole is an antithyroid drug, one of a class of compounds called thioamides all of which were derived from thiourea ('Chemistry and physiology', below). Their antithyroid action was first discovered (1941) when a related chemical, phenylthiourea, was being used to study the sense of taste in rats. Other drugs of this class in clinical use include carbimazole and propylthiouracil. Certain sulphonamides (q.v.) and drugs related to them also have antithyroid action, but the substance longest in use for this purpose is iodine.

Therapeutic use

The antithyroid drugs are used to treat overactivity of the thyroid gland, hyperthyroidism. This condition usually manifests itself in enlargement of the gland, called goitre, although goitre may also appear in the reverse situation, hypothyroidism. In the former, the thyroid appears to produce too much thyroid hormone, while in the latter, too little is produced but the gland may nevertheless enlarge in an apparent response to the demand for normal supplies of the hormone. Other signs of hyperthyroidism include excessive production of body heat, increased excitability of nerves and muscles, insomnia, excessive movement, anxiety, apprehension, increased frequency of bowel movements, softening of the bones due to calcium loss and in some cases, visibly bulging eyes. These latter symptoms may occur without goitre, and are then caused by over-secretion of hormone by a part of the gland. Methimazole appears to be equally effective in all cases.

The causes of hyperthyroidism are unknown. In some cases, it appears suddenly, and may disappear after suitable treatment. Perhaps fifty per cent of patients who receive antithyroid drugs eventually recover completely, though the drugs do not themselves cure the condition. Chemotherapy is indeed often used prior to radiation therapy, by means of radioactive iodine, and surgery to remove part of the gland.

Speculation on the cause of hyperthyroidism now canvasses the possibility that the illness is an auto-immune disease; that is, one in which cells that normally produce antibodies against foreign invaders such as bacteria and viruses begin instead to synthesize antibodies which attack the tissues of the body itself (see 'Azathioprine' and 'Indomethacin'), in this case the hormone-producing cells of the thyroid gland. A chemical tentatively named Long-acting Thyroid Stimulator (LATS) has been found in the blood of hyperthyroid patients. It acts differently from thyrotropin, the thyroid-stimulating hormone (q.v.) secreted by the pituitary, and it appears to bear a resemblance to the antibody-carrying substance, gamma-globulin, a blood-borne protein. If LATS is implicated in the occurrence of hyperthyroidism, the antithyroid drugs may mitigate the effects of the damage done by the aberrant antibodies, but cure would be possible only if the responsible cells ceased to produce them.

Side effects

These are infrequent, affecting about seven per cent of patients who receive methimazole. The proportion is even lower with propylthiouracil and slightly higher with carbimazole. However, those which occur can very rarely include a serious blood disorder called agranulocytosis. A mild skin rash is the most common side effect, and some patients experience pain and stiffness in joints, particularly in hands and wrists. Nausea, gastrointestinal upset and headaches have also been reported.

Chemistry and physiology

The thyroid gland, at the base of the neck, produces a hormone (q.v.) which affects the behaviour of almost all body tissues. In its presence, metabolism (q.v.) and growth are within normal ranges. Hyperthyroidism is characterized by signs of gross overstimulation ('Therapeutic use', above), and in the absence of the hormone, growth is impaired and weakness, lassitude, general debility and death may ensue.

The thioamides all contain a carbon atom linked to two nitrogen atoms on one side, and to a sulphur atom opposite to them:

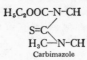

Methimazole   Carbimazole   Propylthiouracil

The actions of these chemicals are in fact unclear. It is most likely that they either inhibit an enzyme (q.v.) involved in the iodination of tyrosine molecules, or they prevent formation of iodide ion from iodine. The process of iodination is known to occur even in the presence of the drugs, though at a much reduced rate. The evidence with respect to the ionization of iodine is less clear.

Methotrexate

(Y. Subba Row, *et al.*, 1948, U.S.) Trade name: none. Administration: oral, in tablets, or by injection.

Classification

Methotrexate is a tissue-destroying drug, correctly called cytotoxic or cell-poisoning, as are actinomycin D (q.v.), azathioprine (q.v.), chlorambucil (q.v.) and 5-fluorouracil (q.v.). Its antimetabolic action (see 'Metabolism'; 'Chemistry and physiology', below) differs from the others, however, in that it prevents the normal use of the vitamin (q.v.), folic acid, by cells. It was the first drug which produced a reversal of the symptoms (remission) for a short time in acute leukaemia of children.

Therapeutic uses

Methotrexate is still used in the treatment of acute leukaemia in children, though when used alone it produces remissions of up to a few months in only about half of the patients who have received it. Better results are obtained when the compound is administered in combination with vincristine, 6-mercaptopurine and prednisone (the two former are also anti-metabolites, and the latter is a steroid – see 'Hormone'), or prednisolone (similar to prednisone).

Far greater success, amounting in fact to cure, has been achieved with methotrexate in the treatment of a rare form of cancer, choriocarcinoma, which occurs in relation to pregnancy. However, this very nearly unique achievement stems as much from the availability of a sensitive test for the presence of the disease as from the drug itself. The urine of women with choriocarcinoma contains excessive amounts of a substance which is normally present. The tumour cells produce the excess, so that the drug can be given in a short series of doses, the test applied to determine whether any cancer cells remain, and so on.

Methotrexate has also been used with moderate success to treat Burkitt's lymphoma (a malignancy found largely in children in tropical Africa, distinguished by the fact that it too can apparently be cured), breast, cervical and vaginal cancer, cancer of the throat and neck, and (with chlorambucil and actinomycin D) testicular cancer. It is of limited value against leukaemia in adults.

Psoriasis is a non-malignant but disturbing and unsightly skin disease characterized by excessive growth of surface cells (see 'Fluocinolone acetonide'). Its causes are unknown, but methotrexate has been useful in controlling it.

Side effects

Like other anti-metabolites, methotrexate can damage or kill normal as well as diseased cells. Its usefulness depends on the more rapid growth and division of cells in some, though by no means all, malignancies. However, those body tissues in which cells also grow rapidly, such as bone marrow and the mucosal lining of the gastrointestinal tract, often suffer toxic effects from the drug. These manifest themselves as disorders of cells in the blood, and as ulcers, bleeding and haemorrhage in the stomach and intestines. Other side effects include diarrhoea, loss of hair, skin rashes, general weakness and loss of appetite. The drug may cause abnormal development of the foetus, and should not be given to women during pregnancy.

Chemistry and physiology

In chemical structure, methotrexate closely resembles the vitamin, folic acid:

Folic acid: R_1=H
R_2=OH

Methotrexate: R_1=CH$_3$
R_2=H

This similarity allows methotrexate to compete with folic acid for the binding site on an enzyme (q.v.), folate reductase, which normally converts the vitamin into a substance essential for the biosynthesis of amino acid bases later incorporated into ribonucleic acid (RNA) and deoxyribonucleic acid (DNA). The drug may also inhibit other enzymes along this same biosynthetic pathway. It binds so tightly to folate reductase, however, that the inhibition of this enzyme is all but irreversible.

Sooner or later resistance to the drug action manifests itself as tolerance for the agent. That is, the cancer cells themselves no longer are damaged or killed by it. It is thought that this resistance develops because sensitive cells die off leaving those which are less subject to the drug action. The difference in the degree of sensitivity would have to be a genetic inheritance of the respective cells. There could be two mechanisms by which this insensitivity might manifest itself: resistant cells may produce excessive amounts of the enzyme, folate reductase, so that some molecules of the enzyme are left free to bind normally and reversibly with folic acid, or resistant cells may possess membranes which differ in some manner so that they are able to exclude the drug. The greater success of treatments which combine methotrexate with other compounds ('Therapeutic uses', above) probably stems in part from the fact that the malignant cells do not become resistant to the other agents at the same time.

The mechanism of action of methotrexate against psoriasis is unknown.

Methyldopa

(Oates, *et al.*, 1960, U.S.) Trade names: Aldomet, Hydromet (with hydrochlorothiazide). Administration: oral, or by injection.

Classification

Methyldopa is chemically related to L-Dopa (q.v.) and adrenaline (q.v.). It is classed as an adrenergic blocking agent; that is, it acts at least in part by impairing the normal functions of nerves which transmit impulses from fibre to fibre or from nerve to muscle by means of the chemical, noradrenaline ('Chemistry and physiology', below). Other drugs of this class include guanethidine (q.v.), bretylium and reserpine.

Therapeutic uses

The principal use of methyldopa is to control abnormally high blood pressure (hypertension; see 'Chlorothiazide'). The compound is most effective against moderate hypertension, although it is used also in severe cases and against sudden rises in blood pressure called hypertensive crises. It acts in about two hours, reaching a peak in four to six hours and continuing to show effects up to twenty-four hours. If thiazides, such as chlorothiazide (q.v.), are being given, the two agents may be administered together, but guanethidine and reserpine are not usually continued if therapy with methyldopa is begun. These drugs may not cure hypertension but, in some cases, blood pressure will become easier to control after use of the agents, or may even return to a normal level when they are discontinued.

Methyldopa has also been moderately useful in treatment of two rare forms of tumour, carcinoid disease (a tumour of the small intestine, stomach, appendix or colon), and phaeochromocytoma, a growth in the adrenal gland, one of the symptoms of which is high blood pressure.

Side effects

During the first two or three days, the drug causes drowsiness, but this usually disappears unless larger doses are given. The agent will cause a sudden fall in blood pressure on standing erect (postural hypotension) or, rarely, after exercise, but less severe than that produced by guanethidine. Other side effects can occasionally include depression and psychic effects, nightmares, nausea, dryness of the mouth, nasal stuffiness, gastrointestinal upset, diarrhoea and constipation, failure of ejaculation, fever and dizziness. Less frequently, headache, the build-up of excess body fluids (oedema), lactation, skin rash, weakness and aggravation of angina pectoris may occur, and rarely, reversible blood disorders and liver damage and an occasional case of Parkinson's disease have also been reported after the use of methyldopa. It should be noted that the urine may darken after the drug is taken.

Patients with liver disease, kidney disorders or a history of mental depression should not be given methyldopa.

Chemistry and physiology

The compound is a catecholamine (see 'Adrenaline'), and chemically similar to dopa, a normal precursor of noradrenaline, and of another chemical transmitter of nervous impulses between neurons, 5-hydroxytryptamine (5-HT, serotonin, see 'Phenelzine'). Its mode of action is uncertain, but because of its structural similarity to dopa, it is thought that it may compete with that substance for an enzyme (q.v.), dopa decarboxylase, which then converts methyldopa to a distorted form of dopamine and of noradrenaline, methylnoradrenaline. This substance is sufficiently similar to natural noradrenaline so that neuronal transmission which depends on noradrenaline can continue, though less efficiently.

The degree of contraction of peripheral blood vessels which contribute to the regulation of blood pressure is controlled by adrenergic nerves. Thus, the milder postural hypotension ('Side effects', above) would be explained by the mode of action described. Central nervous effects such as depression might arise because of disturbances in the biosynthesis of 5-HT. The usefulness of methyldopa in treatment of carcinoid tumour and phaeochromocytoma is also thought to stem from its inhibition of dopa decarboxylase, though the connexion between this chemical action and control of the tumours is not clear.

Metronidazole

(Cosar and Julou, 1959, Fr.) Trade names: Flagyl, Clont (Ger.), Trichazol (Can.). Administration: oral, or as vaginal pessaries.

Classification
One of a class of chemical compounds called nitro-imidazoles ('Chemistry and physiology', below) developed to counter infections by a unicellular organism, *Trichomonas*, categorized as a protozoan.

Therapeutic uses
Trichomoniasis may be accompanied by diarrhoea and debility, and it causes severe vaginal discharge, and infection of the male urethra and bladder. Like so many protozoal infections, including malaria (see 'Mepacrine') and schistosomiasis, this disease is endemic in tropical countries and relatively less frequent though by no means rare in temperate regions with high sanitary standards. Although infection is common to both sexes, symptoms of the disease appear more frequently in women. Metronidazole kills *Trichomonas* rapidly in most patients. Reinfection of women occurs during sexual intercourse, however, and in such circumstances simultaneous treatment of the male partner with the drug is necessary, even though he may be without symptoms.

The drug has proved to be useful against giardiasis, also a

protozoal infection, and against an unpleasant and painful condition of the gums called Vincent's infection. It may serve as a urinary antiseptic against certain types of bacteria which can infect the genito-urinary tract.

Side effects

These are rarely severe. Evidence of gastrointestinal upset is most common. Occasional headache and vomiting, and, rarely, central nervous disturbances may occur. Itching, flushing, pelvic pressure and dryness of the mouth, vagina and vulva have been reported. Serious blood disorders have not been reported, but a moderate fall in white blood cells occurs occasionally, and should be carefully watched for; withdrawal of the drug is accompanied by a return to normal. Drug metabolites darken the urine.

Metronidazole should not be given to patients with blood disorders or active neurological disease, and probably not to pregnant women.

Chemistry and physiology

The molecule is extremely simple:

$$\begin{array}{c} \text{H-C-N} \\ \text{O}_2\text{N-C-N} \\ \text{CH}_2\text{CH}_2\text{OH} \end{array} \text{C-CH}_3$$

It is believed that the fall in white blood cells may be related to the presence of the nitro (NO_2) group, but its mechanism of anti-protozoal action is unknown.

Morphine

(Sertürner, 1803, Ger.) Administration: injection, oral.

Classification

The principal active constituent of opium, the juice of a poppy plant, *Papaver somniferum*, morphine (named for Morpheus, god of dreams) is the first and still the most widely used opiate. The opiates are also known as narcotic analgesics (pain killers that tend to produce sleep). Codeine is also a natural derivative of opium. It is much weaker than morphine. Heroin, the popular name of diacetylmorphine, is a semi-synthetic compound derived from morphine and stronger than the natural drug. There are a growing number of wholly synthetic opiates with varied strengths and values, developed largely because of the search for a non-addictive drug with the therapeutic usefulness of morphine. They include methadone (Physeptone; U.S.: Adanon, Dolphine), pethidine (U.S.: meperidine); (Pamergan, Pethilorfan; U.S.: Demerol), and pentazocine (Fortral; U.S.: Talwin). Pentazocine is also a narcotic antagonist, a substance that acts by antagonizing the effects of morphine and other opiates. It is chemically related to nalorphine (nalorphine hydrobromide – Lethidrone; U.S.: nalorphine hydrochloride – Nelline), also a narcotic antagonist (see 'Chemistry and physiology', below).

Therapeutic uses

The Canadian physician, Sir William Osler, described morphine as 'God's own medicine'. It is still the most effective analgesic known for control of chronic pain. Only heroin may be more effective on a weight basis against the acute pain of terminal cancer. So effective are the opiates that it is an old medical rule never to give them before the diagnosis is made because the comfort they bring may dissipate the patient's symptoms. The sedation and tranquillity produced by opiates make them excellent preanaesthetic medication to relax the patient before surgery, although phenobarbitone (q.v.) may be just as effective without opiate-induced side effects. Opiates can control a persistent cough, but non-narcotic agents are now commonly preferred because of the danger of addiction even to codeine. Morphine may relieve certain breathing difficulties coincident upon heart or lung disease, and opium itself is useful for the treatment of diarrhoea.

Side effects

All known opiates are addictive. The doctor who prescribes them for the control of chronic pain must always select the weakest compound and the lowest dose consistent with relief. Tolerance to the drugs requires that the patient be given larger doses of stronger compounds, and tolerance to one opiate extends to all the others. Once there is a tolerance to them, furthermore, withdrawal of the drugs causes severe physiological disturbances and psychological craving. Morphine and heroin withdrawal symptoms may begin with perspiration, yawning and eye watering followed by restless sleep. Appetite declines, the pupils dilate and the addict becomes increasingly irritable. As these symptoms increase in severity, weakness, nausea, diarrhoea and depression appear. Heart rate and blood pressure rise. The skin is clammy and covered by gooseflesh, the origin, incidentally, of the expression 'cold turkey' for drug withdrawal without support. Cramps and pains develop along with muscle spasms followed by the kicking movements that gave rise to the expression, 'kicking the habit'. In both men and women, spasms may lead to orgasm. Biochemical changes affect breathing and urine content, and these changes in turn disturb the acid-base balance of body fluids. White blood cell count may rise sharply. In extreme cases, there is fatal cardiovascular collapse. Methadone and codeine withdrawal symptoms are usually less severe, but they may spread over a longer time. Narcotic antagonists such as nalorphine will produce withdrawal symptoms if they are given to an opiate addict.

Though tolerance and addiction may be the most serious side effects, more immediate undesirable reactions may also disturb the patient. Nausea, dizziness, mental clouding, constipation and disturbances associated with liver function are common. Many patients experience dysphoria rather than the euphoria for which the opiates are used illegally, and increased sensitivity to pain when the drug effect wears off is also common. Allergic reactions, delirium and insomnia rather than sedation have been noted, though infrequently. Perhaps the most serious immediate side effect is the respiratory depression produced by morphine. Along with coma and pinpoint pupils, it is the most prominent sign of acute morphine poisoning. Blood pressure and body temperature fall, as does the rate of urine formation, and shock and convulsions ensue. They can be fatal. The treatment of choice for acute morphine poisoning is a narcotic antagonist like nalorphine.

Barbiturates (see 'Phenobarbitone') and alcohol (see 'Ethyl alcohol'), both depressant drugs with narcotic effects, hasten and exacerbate the symptoms of morphine poisoning. Anti-depressants (see 'Imipramine', 'Phenelzine') may actually enhance the depressant effect of opiates. Phenothiazines (see 'Chlorpromazine') used to control psychoses increase the sedative effect of opiates but reduce their usefulness as pain-killers. The analgesic value of codeine is greatly increased when it is given with aspirin (q.v.).

Chemistry and physiology

Morphine neither eliminates the psychological perception of pain nor does it halt the sensation. The patient knows that the pain continues, but he is not disturbed by it. The associated fear and tension subside so that the pain becomes bearable. Relief is accompanied by a comfortable drowsiness and often by euphoria. These reactions indicate that the drug works in the central nervous system, particularly in the brain. There is no indication that the drug alters the activity of sensory nerves, in the skin for example, or of peripheral nerves that conduct messages to and from the brain.

The biophysical mechanisms of action are not known. Broadly speaking, the attempt to understand them follows two related lines of research: biochemical changes caused by the drugs, and the molecular sites in the membranes of nerve cells where such changes occur. Both lines of research focus attention on the synapse, the juxtaposed endings of two nerve cells where they are separated by a tiny gap.

Biochemical research has concentrated on the chemical transmitters, molecules that carry a nervous signal across the synaptic gap from a nerve cell to its immediate neighbour. In the periphery, transmitters also carry nervous signals from a nerve cell to a muscle cell or a cell in a gland. The opiates can be shown to alter the synthesis, release and metabolic breakdown (see 'Metabolism') of at least four such chemicals: acetylcholine (ACh), noradrenaline, 5-hydroxytryptamine (5-HT) and dopamine, all of which are believed to act as transmitters in different parts of the brain. There is some positive relationship, moreover, between the observed therapeutic effectiveness of the respective opiates and the degree of change they induce in the concentrations or activity of the transmitters. These changes appear to be most evident in the limbic system, a section of the brain associated with emotion and feelings of pleasure and pain. Drug control of pain as well as the euphoria produced by these compounds might arise because of their actions in the limbic system, but the respiratory depression caused by opiates must involve other brain centres.

Biochemical changes affecting the transmitters could also explain physiological aspects of withdrawal and tolerance. For example, if the drug impairs the function of acetylcholine (ACh), an enzyme (q.v.) required for synthesis of new ACh may be stimulated. More of the drug will be required to inhibit the increased supply of ACh. But if the drug is withdrawn, the inhibition disappears and the more rapid synthesis continues, intensifying the normal effects of the transmitter. The evidence for such connexions is contradictory and inconclusive, but disturbance of transmitter metabolism could explain the actions of the opiates.

There is also evidence that morphine inhibits an action by prosta-glandins (q.v.) which could alter the behaviour of nerve cells. The inhibition would reduce protein synthesis by nerve cells, and there is some independent evidence that opiates have such an effect. Although the transmitter chemicals are not proteins, enzymic proteins are re-quired for their synthesis and breakdown. No relation has yet been established, however, between the reduction of protein synthesis and the putative changes in the concentration or activity of the transmitters.

These chemicals act when their molecules attach to molecules in the membranes of the post-synaptic nerve cell. (For description of ACh receptor, see 'Atropine'.) There is indirect evidence that the opiates may also act by attaching to receptor molecules normally intended to receive the transmitters. The problem is to determine the structure and normal function of these receptors. The opiates comprise a varied class of chemicals which produce similar effects. Either there is a common structure hidden within the molecules of the respective opiates that has not yet been discovered, or the different opiates attach to different receptors, or possibly both.

The narcotic antagonists (see 'Classification', above) are thought to compete with opiates for the receptor molecules on nerve cell mem-branes. The competition cannot be quite so straightforward, however, because most antagonists exhibit some opiate-like activity too. For example, nalorphine and pentazocine are also effective pain-killers. Indeed, pentazocine is a mild antagonist with important uses as a morphine substitute. The drug appears to be less addictive than morphine, and tolerance to it develops more slowly. Complex models have been suggested to explain the contradictory activities of narcotic antagonists by describing a sequence of events at putative receptors, but none of them has yet been demonstrated. Meanwhile, the search continues for a drug with the analgesic power of morphine but with-out its addictive side effect.

Neostigmine

(Aeschlemann and Reinert, 1931, Ger.) Trade name: Pros-tigmin. Administration: injection, oral or by direct application in liquid to the eye.

Classification

A synthetic drug closely related chemically to a natural derivative of the Calabar or ordeal bean (*Physostigma venenosum*), physo-stigmine or eserine, from which it was developed. Other similar agents include pyridostigmine, benzpyrinium, demecarium and ambenonium. Neostigmine is thus one of a class of moderately 'reversible' anticholinesterase agents; i.e. drugs which inhibit an enzyme (q.v.), cholinesterase, and thus allow the persistence in tissue of acetylcholine (see 'Atropine'), a transmitter of nerve impulses between nerve ends and between nerves and muscles in the voluntary nervous system and in parts of the para-sympathetic division of the autonomic (involuntary) nervous system. Two other classes of inhibitors exist: rapidly 'reversible', exemplified by edrophonium, and poisonous, 'irreversible' inhibitors which include many insecticides and poison gases ('Chemistry and physiology', below).

Therapeutic uses
The peristaltic movement of the small intestine, which moves partially digested food from the duodenum near the junction with the stomach to the large intestine, is produced by muscles under involuntary nervous control. Either because of disease or as a result of surgery, the normal movement of these muscles may be interrupted; they become partially or wholly paralysed, a condition called paralytic ileus. Neostigmine is the most frequently used of this class of drugs to correct or prevent paralytic ileus, although employment of the compound is often in addition to some physical therapy such as suction. The drug is not used if the bowel is obstructed, or when infection is present.

Surgery can also produce abnormal constriction of the sphincter muscles which control release or retention of urine by the bladder. Neostigmine serves to relax these muscles.

Although its mechanism of action may be quite different in the achievement of this end, the compound is also valuable in restoration of muscular tone when the patient suffers from a disease called myasthenia gravis. The condition reveals itself in weakness and abnormally rapid tiring of the skeletal muscles, those in the arms, legs and face, for example, which are under voluntary nervous control. The cause of the disease is unknown, however, and the drug corrects the symptoms without curing the underlying factors. It is worth noting that in a normal patient, by contrast, neostigmine produces some reduction in muscle tone.

Used in the eye, the agent lowers muscular resistance to the outflow of the fluid which normally fills the eyeball. This action is of great value in the treatment of glaucoma, an abnormal increase in the amount of intraocular fluid which builds up pressure inside the eye and can lead to irreversible blindness.

Side effects

Neostigmine has fewer side effects than physostigmine or other drugs of its class, but poisoning can occur if the agent is given for a prolonged period or in large doses. The symptoms of poisoning include restlessness, weakness, nausea, vomiting, possibly diarrhoea, abdominal pain and, rarely, abnormal relaxation of the eye muscles. These events may be followed by salivation, sweating, weeping, palpitation and slowed pulse, shortness of breath, muscular twitching and convulsions. Atropine (q.v.) is the most effective antidote to neostigmine poisoning. Neostigmine should be given only with the greatest caution to patients with asthma, certain forms of heart disease, low blood pressure, parkinsonism or epilepsy.

Chemistry and physiology

The molecular mechanism of action of neostigmine and related drugs has been thoroughly investigated. Though it is, therefore, remarkably well understood, the physiological effects of the drugs are so complex that the effort to unravel and relate them to its actions at the molecular level provides an excellent insight into the connexion between modern biology and medicine.

The drug molecule is called an ammonium–carbamyl ester:

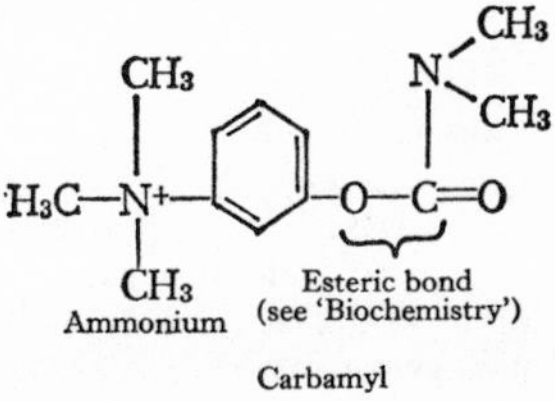

It bears an important structural resemblance to acetylcholine (ACh; see 'Atropine'):

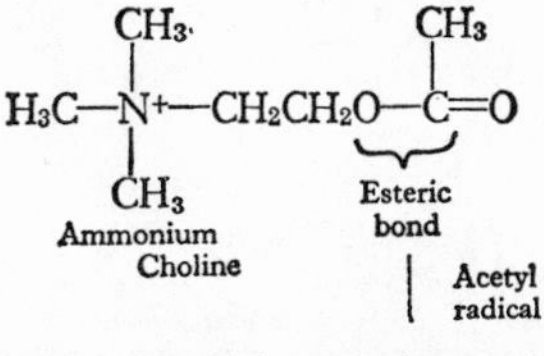

Acetylcholine is the chemical transmitter which carries nerve impulses between the nerves of parts of the parasympathetic system and the involuntary muscle cells it regulates, between nerves in certain autonomic ganglia (i.e., nerve junction boxes outside the brain and spinal cord), and between voluntary nerves and the muscle cells in the voluntary, skeletal muscles. When a nerve impulse passes along a cholinergic nerve, ACh is released from the nerve end in order to transmit the impulse to another nerve or to a muscle cell. In the intercellular space at the nerve end, however, there is an enzyme, acetylcholinesterase (AChE), the function of which is to inactivate ACh. The enzyme acts very quickly so that, under normal circumstances, the ACh is neutralized in time to allow the next nerve in line or the muscle cell to return to its resting state before another nerve impulse releases another quantum of ACh, and the process is repeated.

The enzyme molecule (AChE) catalyses the breakdown of the transmitter molecule (ACh) because it binds ACh at two points. The positively charged ammonium moiety becomes attached to a negatively charged site on the enzyme, and the acetyl moiety is thereby brought into contact with another, positively charged enzymic site. When the esteric bond is broken by further chemical reaction between enzyme and substrate (the substance on which the enzyme works, in this case ACh), the acetyl remains momentarily attached to the enzyme while the choline is released. Thereupon, the acetyl-enzyme complex is hydrolysed (see 'Biochemistry'), and the acetyl is in turn released as a molecule of acetic acid.

The similar structure of neostigmine allows it to be bound by the enzyme at the same two enzymic sites as is ACh. Again the enzyme breaks the esteric bond, releasing the ammonium moiety, but the carbamyl portion of the drug molecule remains attached to the enzyme and is far less readily hydrolysed than is the acetyl segment of ACh. For this reason, AChE is immobilized for periods which vary according to the amount of the drug present, and other factors.

When AChE is put out of action by neostigmine, it can no longer inactivate ACh. The continued presence of the transmitter prevents relaxation of the nerve or muscle cell so that a condition of permanent excitation or contraction, called tetany in muscles, can ensue. This appears to be what happens when the drug is used to treat myasthenia gravis. Because excitation causes the relevant muscles of the eye to relax rather than to contract, furthermore, preservation of intercellular ACh permits drainage of intraocular fluid and combats glaucoma.

The structural resemblance between ACh and neostigmine causes the drug to have a second mode of action. ACh transmits nervous impulses because after its release by the 'initiating' neuron, it combines with a receptor molecule on the 'following' neuron or muscle cell (see 'Atropine'). Neostigmine may also attach itself to those receptors, but if it does, the nerve or muscle cell is inactivated. This probably explains the weakness and muscle twitch among other symptoms of anti-AChE drug-poisoning.

Finally, when they are suitably stimulated, some non-nervous tissues, particularly portions of the intestine, release ACh as a local hormone (q.v.). Again, neostigmine prevents the neutralization of

ACh by AChE. In part at least it is this action which enhances the usefulness of the agent for treatment of paralytic ileus.

These various actions can of course be contradictory. The drug both tends to slow heart rate and to relax muscles which constrict small blood vessels, leading to a fall in blood pressure. But the ganglionic effects of the drug first tend to emphasize and then to contradict the cardiovascular effects. Accumulation of ACh, furthermore, contributes to constriction of the bronchial tubes (thus the drug is contraindicated for asthmatics; 'Side effects', above); this and other actions create an oxygen shortage which by reflex action tends to speed up the heart.

Oestradiol

(Synthesized: Butenandt, *et al.*, 1937, Ger.) Also: Estradiol. Trade names: Natural compounds of various chemical forms: Primogyn Depot, Hormonin, Primosiston, Micryston Oestrone, Ovestin, Premarin; synthetic compounds in various chemical forms: Estrovis, Pentovis, Vallestril, Lynoral, Primogyn C, Amenorone, Menstrogen, Pregornot, Anovlar 21, Controvlar, Norlestrin, Primodos; synthetics with various sedatives or tranquillizers and other compounds: Barboestril, Equadiol, Menopax, Oestrad, Oestradin, Climatone, Femipausin, Mepilin, Mixogen, Primodian, Secrodyl, Tova. Administration: oral, injection and implantation.

Classification
The most active of the naturally occurring female hormones (q.v.), originally isolated as a group from pregnancy urine, and subsequently separated into individual components. Oestradiol is almost inactive when taken by mouth; modifications of the molecule have led to the development of various compounds, e.g. ethinyl oestradiol, mestranol, which refine activity when they are taken by mouth. Certain non-steroidal compounds which are also highly active orally have been developed, including the first, diethylstilboestrol (stilboestrol), and related substances such as hexoestrol and benzestrol. Related compounds are quinestrol, methallenoestrol, oestradiol valerate, chlortrianisone, and dinoestrol.

Therapeutic uses
Despite the wide variety of preparations available, the therapeutic uses of oestrogens in terms of disease entities treated are

relatively limited. The most extensive use is in the oral contraceptive (discussed under 'Progesterone'), and there is an increasing use in the treatment of the upsets of the menopause, particularly in the U.S.A., the menopause being that time of life in the female when ovarian function decreases and body levels of oestrogen decrease. At this time too certain body tissues, for example the vagina and vulva, which are responsive to the blood levels of oestrogen may become dry and liable to infection. Such conditions respond well to the local application of oestrogen-containing creams. Similar preparations have been advocated for bust development but there is no evidence that they produce improvement which cannot be obtained by oral tablets, nor that side effects of effective doses are any less. Also at the time of the menopause a form of arthritis which may occur has been ascribed to oestrogen deficiency. Although many rheumatologists resist the suggestion, the fact that the disease responds to oestrogen therapy suggests that this is the primary causative factor.

The hormone may be used for treatment of acne in pubertal girls and sometimes later. The condition can be strikingly relieved, presumably due to the action of the administered preparation (usually oral contraceptives) to diminish sebum (skin oil) production. Hirsutism, which in some cases appears to be due to excess androgen production from the adrenal gland (see 'Hormones'), may be suppressed via the feedback mechanism to the pituitary by the administration of oestrogen-containing preparations. Some physicians consider such uses to be cosmetic only.

Because women suffer from heart attacks less frequently than men, oestrogen has also been suggested for their prevention in men. When oestrogen levels decrease after the menopause, the frequency of heart attacks is more nearly the same in both sexes. Unfortunately most trials of oestrogen as a prophylactic in men have not been successful, and have been associated with a high incidence of undesirable side effects, for example breast enlargement and loss of libido.

Perhaps the most striking efficacy of oestrogen-containing preparations in gynaecology has been seen in their use in dysmenorrhoea (painful periods) for which they are usually given cyclically starting five days after a menstrual period and continuing for twenty to twenty-one days, often in the form of an oral contraceptive. Their mode of action in bringing about relief in these cases is not certain, but there is strong evidence to indicate that it is by inhibition of ovulation.

Apart from their use in straightforward ovarian deficiency, oestrogens have two further main applications: in the treatment of prostatic carcinoma in the male, and in the amelioration of breast cancer in the female. While the rationale for their use in the former is reasonably clear (presumably an opposition to the stimulating effect which the male hormone testosterone has on the cancer cells), it is less easy to understand why this type of compound should be effective in the latter where one is dealing with a disease which is thought to be dependent on oestrogen for its growth and that, indeed, responds favourably to removal of the ovaries – the main source of oestrogen in the body. However, if one examines the basis for the claim that oestrogens are effective against breast cancer, it becomes clear that the more effective the oestrogenic compound in treating the disease, the less closely related it is in chemical structure to oestradiol. Thus compounds such as stilboestrol (perhaps the most effective 'oestrogen' in this condition) which is not even steroidal in structure may be acting as blockers of access to the cancer cells by oestradiol so that they have no access to the natural hormone which they require for growth and cell division. Certainly this would explain the greater efficacy of such compounds as drostanolone propionate (an anti-oestrogen) in treating this disease.

Side effects

Few side effects are associated with the administration of oestrogens, either orally or by injection. By far the most common is nausea, and very occasionally vomiting or diarrhoea, the nausea being similar to that seen in early pregnancy and passing off after a few months' treatment. Fluid retention, breast engorgement and irritability have also been blamed on oestrogen administration, and, rarely, allergy which takes the form of an overall rash may occur. Certain metabolic alterations are also known to occur, in the shape of diminution of carbohydrate tolerance (the ability of the body to handle a sudden load such as occurs after a meal), alterations in blood fat levels, and alterations in the level of various factors in the blood concerned with clotting (see 'Heparin') and occasionally of liver function, particularly in Swedish women who appear to be excessively intolerant to oestrogens. So far these changes, which have been studied mainly in women on oral contraceptives, but which appear on present evidence to be associated with the oestrogen component, have been observed to be entirely reversible, and it is doubtful whether they are of any long-term significance. One side effect which is of relatively minor importance in terms of incidence despite its statistical significance, is thrombosis (see 'Progesterone' for a discussion of the relative risks of this occurrence). It appears possibly to be related to certain biochemical changes, particularly those concerned in blood clotting (above). Thrombosis has been seen both in women on oral contraceptive preparations containing oestrogen, and in men being treated for cancer of the prostate with stilboestrol. Indeed in one trial more patients died from thrombosis which may have been associated with the use of oestrogens than from the prostatic cancer itself. None the less because the cancer would ultimately have spread throughout the body, causing unpleasant complications from secondary deposits, the fact that it was held in check by the oestrogens still justifies the use of this form of therapy.

Allegations that oestrogens may cause breast cancer and cancer of other genital organs in the female have frequently precipitated 'scares' in newspapers, due to irresponsible and hysterical reporting. It must be emphasized that all such suggestions are based on animal work using enormous doses (up to two hundred times the human dose) over periods of time corresponding to twenty years or more in women. There is no evidence to justify the transfer of these results to women, and indeed much evidence in certain species at least that they are not transferable.

Chemistry and physiology

The available oestrogens can be divided into two types on the basis of their chemical structure (although physiologically their actions are similar, differing mainly in potency): the steroidal compounds on the one hand, and the non-steroids on the other.

The steroids are all related to oestradiol, although the equine oestrogens, equilin and equilenin (derived from the urine of pregnant mares) are also unsaturated in the B ring (see 'Hormones'). The synthetic compounds ethinyl oestradiol and mestranol are similar in structure to oestradiol except that both have the addition of an ethinyl-group ($CH \equiv C-$) in position 17, and also in the case of mestranol of a methyl ether ($CH_3 - O -$) in position 3, these conferring a degree of protection to the compounds when given orally.

The non-steroids, however, are related to diethylstilboestrol (formula below) differing mainly in the substituents in place of the two ethyl ($C_2H_5 -$) groups. Why such compounds should have oestrogenic activity is uncertain, but it has been suggested that it is related to the distance between the two hydroxyl groups ($HO-$ or $-OH$), that these are the active groups in the molecule, and that this distance is the same in both oestradiol and stilboestrol.

diethylstilboestrol

The sites of production of oestrogens, their stimulation by follicle-stimulating hormone, and the feedback control are discussed under 'Hormone'. Oestradiol is produced cyclically in the female, its concentration being greatest in the first half of the menstrual cycle, decreasing slightly at the time of ovulation (mid-cycle) and showing a second lesser peak in the second half, diminishing sharply about two days before menstruation. If fertilization takes place, however, the levels of oestrogen in the body increase considerably, at least a part of this being produced in the developing foetus so that assessment of the urinary oestrogen levels in pregnancy gives an indication of the viability of the foetus. Decrease in the level of oestrogen, however, is seen after the menopause when ovarian function diminishes.

Physiologically the oestrogens are responsible for the changes which occur in females at the time of puberty, some of which continue thereafter until the menopause, and for that mysterious attribute, femininity. In the periphery of the body (their central action on the hypothalamus and pituitary is covered in 'Hormones') they cause breast development, particularly of the ducts, with associated fat accumulation; pigmentation of the skin of the nipples and surrounding area, the areola; and of the external genitalia. They help to shape the skeleton by affecting the growing ends of the long bones such that the pubertal spurt of growth with subsequent cessation occurs, and they soften the skin. They cause the lengthening of the vagina and enlargement of the uterus (or womb) which occurs at puberty, and also the characteristically distributed growth of pubic and axillary hair.

After the pubertal changes have occurred, and until the menopause (except during pregnancy) the oestrogens appear to function cyclically. Every month particularly during the first half of the menstrual cycle they cause changes which are directed to the preparation of the organs of the body for fertilization and pregnancy. Thus they cause an increase in libido, although this may be more related to androgen (see 'Testosterone' and 'Hormones') production, they cause the vagina to secrete fluid which acts as a lubricant and may also give off a pheromone (natural odour) to attract the male, and they cause changes in the mucus plug at the neck of the womb which make it more receptive to sperm. In addition they cause a thickening of the lining of the womb, the endometrium, to prepare it for the action of progesterone (q.v.) in the second half of the cycle. The breasts may enlarge further, a change which occurs even more forcibly in relation to the high levels of oestrogen during pregnancy, and the woman may experience a general feeling of well-being due to the mild anabolic (see 'Metabolism', and 'Oxymetholone') effect of oestrogen. The reversal of these effects in response to oestrogen deficiency at the menopause, and their reinstitution by appropriate therapy, have already been considered ('Therapeutic uses' above).

At the cellular level oestradiol has been shown to be bound to the nucleus of cells in its target organs, where it appears to stimulate the synthesis of ribonucleic acid (RNA), possibly by increasing the activity of an enzyme (q.v.), RNA-polymerase, although this increased activity may itself be a consequence of enhanced availability of DNA active as template for RNA synthesis (see 'Actinomycin D').

Oxymetholone

(Synthesized: Ringold, *et al.*, 1958, U.S.) Trade names: Anapolon, Anapolon 50, Adroyd, Anadrol; related compounds: Anabolex, Anaprotein, Lysinex, Neodrol, Durabolin, Deca-Durabolin, Dianabol, Primobolan Depot, Nilevar, Orabolin, Orgabolin, Stenediol, Stromba, Winstrol. Administration: oral, injection.

Classification
One of the more active synthetic compounds related to testosterone (q.v.), especially developed to maximize the anabolic

(see 'Metabolism') activity of the natural male hormone (q.v.) and to minimize its virilizing side effects. Other related compounds are stanolone, nandrolone, methanedienone, ethylestrenol, methyl androsteniol, stanozolol.

Therapeutic uses

Anabolics, correctly used, are of value in conditions where there is a need to stimulate tissue growth, particularly protein synthesis, and when it is advisable to counteract the effects of other stimuli (for example, high fever, or operations) which cause the development of a negative nitrogen balance, that is excretion of a greater quantity of nitrogen in the urine and faeces than is taken in in the diet. Regrettably, anabolic steroids have tended to fall into disrepute due to their use by athletes to stimulate muscle development and increase performance, a practice which is now being discouraged by such means as spot checks on urine samples. The test fails in many cases, however, because the changes which occur after the use of anabolic agents persist for months. Thus the athlete can stop using the drugs some hours before the test is made, and the urine sample will be free of incriminating evidence. It is doubly regrettable that because of the adverse publicity surrounding such use, and the reports of undoubted side effects which follow the administration of the enormously high doses employed, doctors should be discouraged from utilizing the considerable advantages presented by these products for the benefit of their patients.

There is, however, also a body of medical opinion which regards the anabolics as being of doubtful therapeutic value. They hold that the beneficial effects of these compounds can just as well be achieved by improvement of diet. Although this may be true, it overlooks the fact that many indications for anabolic therapy are situations where less food is being eaten and appetite is concomitantly reduced. Anabolics will stimulate appetite by some unknown mechanism and increase food intake. Furthermore, these compounds lead to better metabolic use of nitrogen contained in food.

After major injuries, particularly those involving muscle tissue, after surgical operations, during fever or long-drawn-out disease, the body enters a severe state of catabolism (see 'Metabolism') in which nitrogen loss as a consequence of tissue wasting is significant. In these cases administration of an anabolic agent will certainly cause diminished urinary nitrogen loss, and may even convert a negative nitrogen balance to a positive one. Due to their effect in promoting tissue growth, increased rate of healing may be expected; enhancement of the patient's state of well-being, with consequent stimulation of appetite, will lead to further improvement due to increased caloric (including protein) intake.

Catabolism also occurs during administration of corticosteroids (see 'Hydrocortisone'), and anabolic compounds have been shown experimentally to reverse this situation. Yet here again some medical opinion frowns on combined therapy, and prefers to live with the muscle wasting and bony collapse which are among the possible side effects of the long-term use of corticosteroids.

Use of anabolics in mild chronic disease is perhaps less justifiable, however, but weight gains in such conditions have been due to stimulation of appetite by these compounds.

There are two further situations in which anabolics are of undoubted value. The first of these is in chronic kidney failure, in which there is a considerable increase in the level of urea, a breakdown product of protein, in the blood. By stimulating the synthesis of protein in part from blood urea, anabolics can at least temporarily reduce the level of urea, and diminish the frequency with which such patients require dialysis to clear the blood of this impurity.

The second condition is aplastic and/or hypoplastic anaemia, in which the bone-marrow which produces the majority of the cells of the blood (but in this case particularly the red-cell-producing tissue) appears to cease functioning. A review (1959) of the condition, particularly concerned with its common occurrence in children, concluded that it was one of the most hopeless and discouraging in the practice of paediatrics, that patients had to be kept alive with repeated blood transfusions plus a host of other drugs, and that all measures then available produced uniformly poor results. The situation remained static until 1964, when oxymetholone was first used in treating nineteen patients with apparent cure in seventy per cent. Since then there have been a number of trials, some of which have included cases resistant to other hormonal forms of therapy, and it has been uniformly concluded that this compound is a potent bonemarrow stimulant. Perhaps surprisingly, in view of the high doses employed (up to 300 mg per day of a drug normally given in doses of 7·5 to 15 mg daily), there have been few side effects; in particular, no hastening of cessation of bone growth in children (see 'Testosterone') has occurred.

Side effects

The side effects of the anabolics are similar to those of testosterone and its related compounds, except that virilization is rarely severe. Indeed, in normal clinical doses, it does not often occur, though increased dosage, such as may be employed in treatment of breast cancer, can be associated with a significant incidence of this side effect. Certain of the changes which occur in women following the use of higher doses may not be reversible, for example the deepening of the voice, probably due to anatomical changes in the larynx.

Certain of the anabolics can be associated with the development of jaundice. However, so far as is known, the changes are reversible and regress on cessation of treatment. Occasionally excess body fluids develop after administration of these compounds, but diuretics (q.v.) will control the condition.

In high doses anabolics appear to affect the pituitary production of gonadotrophin (see 'Hormones') presumably by operating the negative feedback mechanism. This action explains the embarrassing impotence of some athletes whose muscular physiques derive from the drugs.

Chemistry and physiology

Anabolic steroids are all closely related to testosterone (injectable preparations) or 17-alpha-methyl-testosterone (oral preparations). Various other substitutions on, or alterations of, the molecule are employed to prolong the activity of the drug after administration.

Despite the fact that extensive metabolic studies have been carried out on volunteers and on patients undergoing treatment, little is known about the physiology of the anabolics, except that they cause retention in the body of nitrogen, and of appropriate quantities of other chemicals required for cell synthesis. That they cause retention of calcium is certain, and radioactive tracer studies have shown that this is due to decreased reabsorption of bone; thus their utility in treating the exaggeration of such reabsorption, osteoporosis (loss of bone substance and associated calcium), which occurs in old age, during bed rest and occasionally after the menopause.

The cellular mechanism of action of anabolic agents is not well understood. It has been postulated that at least in aplastic anaemia it may either act as a synergist (a compound which acts together with another) of a hormone, erythropoeitin, which stimulates the cell in the bone marrow that acts as the precursor of the other blood cells, or alternatively that it increases the rate at which this 'stem cell' divides. Certainly it is known that administration of the compound is associated with a decrease in the time spent in the bloodstream (not in the cells) of radioactive iron, suggesting the increased uptake of iron by the bone marrow which would be expected in association with increased red-cell formation.

Penicillin

(Fleming, 1928, U.K.; therapeutic use: Florey, 1939, U.K.)
Trade names: penicillin-G, benzyl penicillin – Conspen, Crystapen, Eskacillin 100 (buffered powder), Falapen (coated tablets), Hyasorb (coated tablets), Pondets, Solupen, Tabillin, Tamporazan Penicillin; penicillin-G plus additional drugs (shown in brackets): Crystamycin (streptomycin), Penbenemid (probenecid), Pendex (hydroxyamphetamine hydrobromide), Soluvone (streptomycin), Tamporazan P.S.S. (sulphanilamide and sulphathiazole). Benzathine penicillin – Dibencil, Penidural; U.S.: Bicillin, Neolin, Permapen; benzathine penicillin plus penicillin-V: Pen-vee-dural. Procaine penicillin – Avloprocil A.S., Distaquaine-G, Eskacillin 200, Lenticillin, Mylipen, Pro-stabillin, Seclopen; U.S.: Abbocillin-DC, Crysticillin, Lento-pen, Premocillin, Wycillin; procaine penicillin plus penicillin-G and streptomycin: Distavone, Seclomycin. For semi-synthetic penicillins, see the end of this entry. Administration: oral – tablets, powder, liquid; injection; other preparations include aerosols, eye-drops, ear-drops, skin creams and ointments and nasal-drops, but these are considered to be of doubtful value. Penicillin is dispensed in units; one unit equals 0·6 micrograms. One milligram equals 1667 units.

Classification
The first antibiotic (q.v.) to be discovered, purified and used clinically. The story of the accidental discovery by Fleming in a culture infected by the mould, *Penicillium notatum*, is familiar. The compound is also produced by certain species of *aspergilli*, but *penicillium chrysogenum* has been most useful commercially.

This is particularly the case with one strain produced from the stem of a mouldy cantaloup. The first clinical trial of penicillin took place in Oxford in early 1941. A city policeman, dying of a mixed staphylococcal–streptococcal infection, was given the available supplies of the drug. He recovered. So great had been the shortage that the dose was augmented by extracting the compound from the urine of other patients on whom it was being tried. An Oxford don is reputed to have described the agent 'as a remarkable substance, grown in bed-pans and purified by passage through the Oxford Police Force'.* Production of usable supplies of the drug was a joint Anglo–American effort undertaken in the United States during World War II.

Benzyl penicillin (penicillin-G) is one of four constituents of the natural mould; but it is the only one in common clinical use. Benzathine penicillin and procaine penicillin are salts (see 'Biochemistry') of benzyl penicillin developed synthetically because they are excreted more slowly and are thus longer-acting than the natural agent.

Therapeutic uses

For all its 'miraculous' attributes, penicillin-G is a narrow-spectrum antibiotic. At the usual dosage levels, it kills only Gram-positive bacteria (see 'Antibiotic'), and high levels are active against some Gram-negative bacteria also. Although some of the newer, semi-synthetic penicillins (below) destroy Gram-negative organisms, none of this family of drugs is effective against viruses, fungus or protozoal infections such as malaria (see 'Mepacrine').

Thus, the drug is the agent of choice against infections caused by pneumococcus. These include pneumonia, empyema – an inflammation of the lung casing with pus accumulation which can accompany and complicate pneumonia, pneumococcal meningitis, infected arthritis, osteomyelitis, acute mastoiditis, inflammation in the heart (endocarditis), peritonitis and infections of the ear and sinuses due to this organism.

Not all streptococcal infections respond equally well to penicillin. Sore throat, scarlet fever, meningitis, pneumonia, acute endocarditis, eye and skin infections, arthritis and osteomyelitis caused by Group A *Streptococcus pyogenes* are most effectively

*Goodman and Gilman, *op. cit.*, p. 1194.

treated. Similar diseases caused by other streptococcal species respond less well or inconsistently.

At first all staphylococcal conditions were quickly controlled by penicillin, but resistance (see below, and under 'Antibiotics') among these organisms, particularly the 'Golden Staph', *Staphylococcus aureus*, has greatly increased the difficulty of treatment. The conditions caused by staphylococcal organisms are legion, and the use of natural penicillin-G to counter them today depends on prior bacteriological tests to determine their sensitivity. Some semi-synthetic penicillins are consistently more effective.

The obverse of the medal is to be seen in the case of infections caused by meningococci, including arthritis and endocarditis. The drug preferred for treatment of these diseases was at first a sulphonamide (q.v.), but the causative organisms developed resistance to this class of agent, and they have increasingly been replaced by penicillin. Gonococcal infections, the most familiar of which is gonorrhoea, also responded promptly to natural penicillin, at first, but again bacterial resistance to the drug has become a serious clinical problem.

Penicillin remains the drug of first choice against syphilis. In fact it has made treatment of the disease so cheap, simple and effective that the condition appears to have lost its ancient terror. Perhaps this explains the increasing incidence of the disease as much as does greater social 'permissiveness'.

Anthrax, rat-bite fever, actinomycosis, meningitis and endocarditis caused by *Listeria*, and a form of erysipelas, as well as other less common diseases, all respond well to natural penicillin-G. In addition, the drug can be used to prevent certain streptococcal infections, in particular those which appear as recurrences of rheumatic fever, gonorrhoea (if it is given within eight hours of contact) and syphilis (if given within a day of exposure). When penicillin prophylaxis is attempted against other conditions, superinfections ('Side effects', below; and under 'Antibiotics') can occur.

Side effects

Penicillin is not toxic to human cells at very high dose levels. The major danger with the drug is hypersensitivity to it. Hypersensitivity reveals itself in a range of allergy-like reactions which can include skin rashes, mouth sores, fever, disorders of the blood and urine, serum sickness, respiratory failure, heart failure and death. Only about three out of every thousand patients who receive the drug orally display any of these symptoms, but two to two and a half per cent of those who receive penicillin-G by injection and up to five per cent of those who receive injections of procaine penicillin have had hypersensitivity reactions. Furthermore, sensitization to the drug can build up so that a second dose will cause much more severe reactions than the first. People with a history of allergic disorders or with any untoward effects from earlier doses should be given the compound only with the greatest caution.

Superinfections can occur after a long course of treatment or very high doses of penicillin. The drug will have killed off sensitive bacteria which normally inhabit the intestinal tract and other tissues, allowing resistant bacteria more nutrients and more 'space' in which to grow. These runaway imbalances can even cause a pellagra-like condition due to destruction of intestinal bacteria which help the absorption of the vitamin (q.v.), nicotinic acid. Other rare untoward effects have included pain at the site of injection, blood clots, gastrointestinal upsets and some nervous disorders.

Chemistry and physiology

The Penicillin-G molecule is as follows:

Side chain (varied to form semi-synthetic penicillins

Site of action of amidase (in *Eschirichia coli*)

Penicillin nucleus (6-aminopenicillanic acid; 6-APA)

Site of action of penicillinase (β-lactamase)

The penicillin nucleus alone lacks pharmacological activity. It must be both structurally whole, however, and include a suitable side chain for the drug to work.

The mechanism of action at the molecular level is not fully understood, but the drug may bind to an enzyme (q.v.), a transpeptidase, which is in the membrane surrounding the bacterial cell, inside the cell wall. In any event, its effect is to inhibit formation of the nucleotides (sugar–phosphate–amino acids) which are an essential structural element in the cell walls of all bacteria.

Bacteria are unicellular organisms, and consist of cytoplasm containing chromosomes, various other functional organelles and molecules such as proteins, ATP and sugars essential to the life of the organism (see 'Biochemistry'). The cytoplasm is enclosed by a membrane as are all cells, but outside the membrane and enclosing it, bacteria build rigid walls. These are protective both in the sense that they provide a first line of defence against the environment, and in the sense that they keep the cell from literally exploding. The bacterial cytoplasm is much more dense than most fluids in which the organism naturally occurs so that it is osmotically out of balance with its surroundings. Without its rigid wall, the membrane will break and the cell contents leak away.

Penicillin kills only those bacteria which are in the process of building cell walls, either when they are newly formed, or when they are about to divide into two daughter bacteria. It has no effect on stabilized organisms. Nor has it an effect on human cells. Its remarkable lack of toxicity arises because mammalian cells lack cell walls of the type formed by bacteria.

Penicillin-resistant bacteria appear to possess one or more of three characteristics not shared by their less fortunate sensitive relatives (on the genetic aspects of resistance, see 'Antibiotic'). *Staphylococcus aureus* and certain other species produce an enzyme, penicillinase (β-lactamase), which breaks the bond in the four-membered ring of the nucleus. Other species produce an amidase, also an enzyme, which breaks the bond between the nucleus and the side chain. This action is confined principally to Gram-negative bacteria ('Therapeutic uses', above), and is of greater concern because it inactivates those semi-synthetic penicillins which are effective against this type of bacteria. The third action displayed by some penicillin-resistant bacteria is much less well defined. It too seems to arise from genetic differences between the resistant and the sensitive strains, but it has to do with non-enzymal mechanisms of the organisms. Whereas the enzymal resistance seems to develop as a result of selection (those organisms less capable of producing penicillinase or amidase are killed by the drug), bacteria displaying the third form of resistance may occur because of mutation or possibly as a result of transfer of 'resistant' genes from other bacteria of the same or *different* species. The mechanism of transfer is unclear, even though the event has been seen with the microscope, but it involves DNA (see 'Biochemistry') called the R-factor which is distinct from the single chromosome of bacteria.

Semi-synthetic penicillins

Natural penicillin-G has a number of shortcomings which have been either specifically mentioned or implied in the preceding

Name (trade names)	Improvements on Penicillin-G	Administration	Therapeutic uses
Phenoxymethyl penicillin (Penicillin V, Apsin VK, Compocillin-VK, Econocil-VK, Econopen V, Crystapen V, Distaquaine V-K, Icipen, Marhacillin V-K, Penavlon V, Penicals, Stabillin V-K; U.S.: Pen-vee, V-cillin)	More stable in stomach acid; better absorbed from intestine.	Oral	As penicillin-G
Phenethicillin (Chenupen, Darcel, Dramcillin-S, Maxipen, Semopen, Syncillin)	More stable in stomach acid; better absorption from intestine.	Oral	'Mildly resistant' *Staph. aureus*
Methicillin (Dimocillin-RT, Staphcillin)	Resistant to penicillinase	Injection	*Staph. aureus* and other resistant organisms
Cloxacillin (Orbenin; U.S.: Tegopen)	Resistant to penicillinase. Acid stable	Oral Injection	*Staph. aureus* and other resistant organisms
Ampicillin (Penbritin, Polycillin)	Acid stable. Inhibits Gram-negative bacteria	Oral Injection	Flu. Intestinal and heart infections, meningitis, typhoid fever, other diseases caused by Gram-negative bacteria
Carbenicillin (Pyopen)	Inhibits Gram-negative bacteria	Injection	Urinary tract infections, infected burns, systemic infections and septicaemia, and as ampicillin

discussion. It is unstable in the acid conditions of the stomach, rapidly excreted via the kidneys, susceptible to inactivation by penicillinase, ineffective against Gram-negative bacteria except at high tissue levels, conducive to hypersensitivity reactions, and in addition, it penetrates poorly into spinal fluid. Once the drug nucleus had been isolated in the laboratory (1957), it was possible by the addition of different side chains to create new drugs capable of overcoming one or more of these deficiencies, with the exception of the last two. At least a thousand semi-synthetics have been developed, so-called because the penicillin nucleus itself is derived from the organic mould, while the side chain is added in the laboratory. The table on page 195 lists a few of the clinically more important synthetic penicillins, along with some of their attributes.

Side effects are essentially the same as those experienced with penicillin-G. Whenever its use is possible, furthermore, the natural drug is to be preferred, if only to diminish the risk of induction of penicillin-resistant organisms.

Phenacetin

Trade names: Analgin, Ectodyne, Faivre, Quintas, Refagan (all contain other drugs); 'APC' contains aspirin, phenacetin and caffeine. Administration: oral.

Classification

The first of the so-called 'coal-tar' antipyretics or fever-reducing drugs, acetanilid, was introduced in 1916, but is no longer employed clinically. Phenacetin and acetaminophen (Paracetamol) are the only ones which continue to be used, either as mixtures with aspirin (q.v.), or to treat patients who cannot be given aspirin. They are chemically related to aniline, a dye, and there is evidence that certain poisonous effects of phenacetin ('Side effects', below) arise because a small part of the administered dose may be converted to aniline by the body.

Therapeutic uses

The agent is used primarily to control moderate pain from headache, menstruation, aching joints and neuralgia. It will not control severe pain. Like aspirin, this analgesic effect is also accompanied by antipyresis in patients with a fever but not in normal persons.

Side effects

Acetaminophen is thought to have only very mild and rare side effects, but these may include blood disorders and skin eruptions which can be more common and more serious after the use of phenacetin. For reasons which are unclear, large amounts of the latter drug appear to alter the chemical structure of the oxygen- and carbon dioxide-carrying molecule within red blood cells, haemoglobin, so that a functional anaemia may develop. In higher concentrations, the compound can cause red blood cells to lyse or break apart, creating a haemolytic anaemia. Drug-induced anaemia is frequently accompanied by kidney disorders, although it is now believed that phenacetin may also damage kidney cells directly. In extreme cases, phenacetin poisoning can be fatal. Although prescribed doses are unlikely to affect anyone adversely, great differences do exist in individual reaction to the drug.

Both phenacetin and acetaminophen can be habit-forming. It is thought that a patient deprived of either drug after long usage may show withdrawal symptoms, but none of these reactions, whether psychic or physiological, are considered to be strong or frequent enough to call the drug addictive. The rare cases of euphoria reported probably arise out of respite from pain.

As noted under 'Aspirin' ('Side effects'), it is very doubtful whether mixtures of analgesic compounds improve the pain-relieving qualities of any one of them separately. Such mixtures could contain smaller doses of the respective ingredients, thus possibly reducing their toxic side effects, but on the other hand, over-use of such common mixtures introduces the danger of undesirable effects from any one of the components.

Chemistry and physiology

Both acetanilid and phenacetin are converted metabolically (see 'Metabolism') to acetaminophen. It was originally thought that they exerted their pharmacological actions in the form of acetaminophen, but more recent evidence suggests that phenacetin can be effective even when the formation of acetaminophen is inhibited by use of another drug (diethylaminoethyl diphenylpropylacetate). Aniline may also be a metabolic breakdown product of phenacetin.

The molecular mechanism of action is unknown. The drug probably affects the pain centre in the brain, actually raising the threshold of pain. Similarly, it is believed to lower fever by central action.

Phenelzine

(Synthesized: Chessin, Dubnick, Leeson, Scott, 1959, U.S.) Trade names: Nardil; French: Nardelzine. Administration: oral.

Classification
One of a heterogeneous class of drugs called monoamine oxidase (MAO) inhibitors (see 'Chemistry and physiology', below). The first, iproniazid (Marsilid) was developed for the treatment of tuberculosis (see 'Isoniazid'), and was accidentally found to produce mood elevation in patients to whom it was given. Isocarboxazid (Marplan) and phenelzine are closely related to iproniazid chemically. Two other MAO inhibitors, tranylcypromine (Parnate) and pargyline (Eutonyl), have slightly different chemical structures.

Therapeutic uses
The MAO inhibitors were among the first drugs found to be useful for the control of depression (see 'Imipramine'). Phenelzine or tranylcypromine may be preferred for forms of depression complicated by phobic anxiety. On the whole, however, the use of these drugs is waning because they can be dangerous in therapeutically effective doses. They are usually reserved for patients who do not respond to other drugs.

All MAO inhibitors can have hypotensive effects, and pargyline is most often used for the control of high blood pressure.

Side effects
These drugs require days or even weeks to exhibit their antidepressant effects, but undesirable reactions may appear much more swiftly. The effect of an overdose given in an attempt to hasten mood elevation can include agitation, hallucinations, jerky muscular movement, high temperature and convulsions. These symptoms of acute poisoning can be controlled with drugs such as barbiturates (see 'Phenobarbitone') that reduce

excitement, but such antidotes must be used with great caution because they can bring on a serious psychotic episode. The best treatment may be physical support for breathing, heart beat, temperature and liquid balances. Acute MAO inhibitor poisoning can produce either high or low blood pressure. The latter is more frequent, and there may be a chronic fall in blood pressure when the patient stands erect. This chronic effect can be corrected by lying down, but it may also be necessary to reduce the dose being given. Acute high blood pressure usually occurs if the MAO inhibitors are taken with tyramine, a chemical found in Cheddar, Camembert and Stilton cheeses, beer, wine, pickled herring, chicken liver, yeast, broad beans, tinned figs and coffee! Drugs such as methyldopa (q.v.) and certain chemicals related to amphetamine (q.v.) and L-Dopa (q.v.) in combination with MAO inhibitors may also cause acute hypertension.

Iproniazid is rarely used today because it has been shown to cause fatal liver damage. The other MAO inhibitors are safer in this respect. Chronic disturbances can also include tremors, insomnia, sweating, agitation, confusion and other symptoms of central nervous disorder. Less serious untoward reactions such as dizziness, vertigo, headache, difficulty in urination, inhibition of ejaculation, weakness, dry mouth, blurred vision and skin rashes have been noted, and constipation is common.

The MAO inhibitors prolong and intensify the depressant effects of barbiturates, ethyl alcohol (q.v.) and opiates (see 'Morphine'), and they should not be given with the tricyclic anti-depressants (see 'Imipramine').

Chemistry and physiology

Phenelzine and the related MAO inhibitors contain a chemical moiety called hydrazine ($H_2N \cdot NH_2$) which is thought to be the effective portion of the molecule, but cannot be administered separately because it is poisonous. Tranylcypromine and similar compounds are non-hydrazines and are related chemically to amphetamine (q.v.).

The mechanism of action of neither type of drug is understood. The name, MAO inhibitor, indicates that the drugs delay or reduce the activity of one or more enzymes collectively called monoamine oxidase. They occur in most body tissue, especially nerves, brain and liver, where a form of the enzyme is bound to the membrane surrounding intracellular organelles called mitochondria, the sites of the final breakdown of food products for the energy storage molecule, ATP (see discussion of oxidative phosphorylation under 'Vitamin', and 'Biochemistry'). Monoamine oxidase plays an important role in the intra-cellular breakdown of noradrenaline, the chemical transmitter which conveys nervous impulses between nerve cells and between nerve cells and muscles in parts of the autonomic nervous system (see 'Adrenaline' and 'Amphetamine'). The enzyme also catalyses the first step in the breakdown of 5-hydroxytryptamine (5-HT), another chemical that is thought to be a transmitter of nerve impulses between nerve cells in parts of the brain. Thus, inhibition of the enzyme should have the effect of increasing amounts of noradrenaline and 5-HT with-in respective nerve endings. The MAO inhibitors do not disrupt the nerve impulse, however, and under their influence the supply of the transmitter substances is actually enhanced. However, these drugs may also inhibit release of the transmitter into the tiny gap between the neurons. They may also alter the activity of other enzymes and other cell structures.

That the drugs do increase tissue levels of noradrenaline and 5-HT has been demonstrated experimentally. Furthermore, their inhibitory action is irreversible; that is, once the molecules of the drug become attached to enzyme molecules (or to receptor molecules located on or in membranes), they are fixed there by strong bonds (see 'Bio-chemistry'), and remain until the enzyme itself is broken down and excreted from the cell. The effects of the drug can only be reversed by the biosynthesis of new enzyme, a process that may take weeks.

However, it remains to demonstrate a connexion between these biochemical changes and the symptoms of depression itself, to say nothing of the mood elevation produced by the drugs. For further dis-cussion of this central point, see 'Imipramine'.

Phenobarbitone. U.S.: Phenobarbital

(Loewe, Juliusburger and Impens, 1912) Trade names: Barbenyl, Gardenal, Luminal; with other drugs: Alepsal, Anirrit, Barbevite, Becosed, Beplete, C.B.L. tablets, Feno-belladine, Imbal, Mawplex-B, Milepsi, Phenomet, Scorbital, Sedalby, Seominal, Tab-sed, Thenotrate, Theo-gardenal, Theominal, Tropenal. Administration: oral, but can be injected.

Classification
Phenobarbitone is the second oldest in a widely used class of synthetic drugs called barbiturates. The first was barbitone (U.S.: barbital; 1902). These two agents are among the long-acting barbiturates (below). Other familiar drugs of this large class in-clude pentobarbitone (short-acting) and thiopentone (very short-acting). Primidone, although not a barbiturate, is closely

related chemically to phenobarbitone with which it may be used in the treatment of epilepsy. All of these drugs depress the central nervous system (CNS).

Therapeutic uses

Because the long-acting barbiturates may not take effect for an hour or more and then continue to act for between six and ten hours, they are not often used as sleeping pills (hypnotics). It is the intermediate (thirty-minute onset, five- or six-hour duration) or short-acting (fifteen-minute onset, two- or three-hour duration) compounds which normally serve this purpose. Some authorities now hold that these durational differences are illusory for most barbiturates and that the method of classification by duration of action is, therefore, meaningless.

Phenobarbitone is used as a hypnotic and a sedative, however, for some patients whose insomnia is of nervous origin. It is more often used as a sedative in anxiety, neuroses which affect the heart and stomach, neurasthenia, menstruational and meno-pausal disorders, hyperthyroidism (see 'Methimazole') and for relief of migraine. It may be employed with other drugs such as theobromine to reduce insomnia associated with high blood pressure.

The agent has special value in the prevention and control of grand mal epilepsy. Rapid withdrawal of phenobarbitone from an epileptic who has used it for some time can induce acute epileptic seizures which may be fatal. The drug may be given with primadone or phenytoin, a non-barbiturate compound, in order to reduce the danger of barbiturate poisoning ('Side effects', below) which must be countered by withdrawal.

Only the very short-acting barbiturates are normally used for anaesthesia or for pre-anaesthetic sedative medication. These agents may also be employed to reduce pain during childbirth. All barbiturates tend to enhance the effects of pain killers.

Side effects

Within the usual dosage ranges, the barbiturates are not toxic. The appearance of symptoms of barbiturate intoxication, which can in extreme cases be fatal, result from overdosage, either accidental or intentional. Much larger amounts of the long-acting compounds such as phenobarbitone than of the short-acting agents are required to produce poisoning, but it should be borne in mind that most sleeping pills are intermediate- or short-acting. However, one of the reasons why the long-acting drugs persist is that they are slowly excreted. It is possible, therefore, to build up a dangerously high level of these compounds in the bloodstream. Evidence suggests, furthermore, that alcohol increases the danger of barbiturate intoxication by decreasing the amount required to produce poisoning.

The symptoms are at first similar to drunkenness, but they progress rapidly to coma. The pupil of the eye is at first constricted and then dilated paralytically. Breathing is increasingly disturbed. Blood pressure falls, the pulse becomes weak and rapid and the patient enters shock. Death most often occurs from respiratory failure when the cause is a short-acting barbiturate, and from pneumonia or a related pulmonary disease and kidney failure if the drug is phenobarbitone or another long-acting agent. Most therapy is physical; e.g. washing out the stomach, tubes and artificial respiration to assist breathing, blood transfusions to avoid the circulatory collapse that accompanies shock and the employment of an artificial kidney. The role of drugs as barbiturate antagonists and stimulants is controversial.

Certain other side effects occur infrequently. These have included allergy-type reactions – most often skin rashes, and disorders of the blood and urine. Patients who prove to be sensitive to the compounds should no longer receive any barbiturates. Prior malfunctions of kidneys or liver, shock or porphyria, a rare blood disease, are also contra-indications.

All barbiturates can be addictive; they tend to create both a physiological and a psychic dependence. The danger of poisoning is greatly increased if any of these agents is injected, the method of self-administration recently favoured by addicts. Withdrawal may produce typical symptoms, and can be fatal if it is too sudden.

Chemistry and physiology

The barbiturates are derivates of urea, one of the most common body wastes, plus another organic compound, malonic acid. Their molecular mechanisms of action are unknown. When the compounds are present, less oxygen is used by the brain, and less heat is produced generally. It is thought that they alter both cellular acquisition and storage of energy, and interfere with utilization of energy which is stored. There is also evidence that the drugs alter the behaviour of the membranes surrounding cells so that the movement of ions (q.v.) into and out of cells is distorted, but the connexion, if any, between these events and the disturbances of energy utilization is unclear. Barbiturates affect the nerve ends throughout the body in such a way that the nerves become less responsive to the chemical transmitter substances (see 'Adrenaline', 'Atropine'). Similarly, the compounds depress receptors of the chemical transmitters which convey nervous impulses from neurons to muscle cells both in the voluntary and the involuntary muscles.

The barbiturates are general depressants. They affect not only the CNS but peripheral nerves, muscle, including heart muscle, and various other tissues. Their actions are in other words quite non-specific, and may be altered both by the condition of the individual and by his normal metabolic processes, including the acid-base balance of his body fluids, his mental state, the efficiency of his liver and his degree of allergy-like sensitivity to the drugs.

Phenoxybenzamine

(Smith Kline and French Laboratories Ltd., 1952, U.S.). Trade names: Dibenyline; U.S.: Dibenzyline. Administration: oral, intravenous injection.

Classification
One of a class of chemicals called haloalkylamines closely related to the poison gas, nitrogen mustard (see 'Chlorambucil'). Phenoxybenzamine is the only one of a large series of compounds which is used clinically. All of these drugs block certain nerve impulses ('Chemistry and physiology', below), and this action is the major source of their usefulness. Tolazoline and phentolamine are both agents which act similarly, though they differ chemically from phenoxybenzamine.

Therapeutic uses
This drug, or phentolamine, is employed to control high blood pressure caused by a tumour in the adrenal gland which is called phaeochromocytoma. The growth is usually removed surgically in order to restore the patient to health, and the drug is useful before and during surgery, as well as in cases where the tumour is for some reason inoperable.

Phenoxybenzamine has also been used to treat disorders of the peripheral blood vessels such as chilblains, and one rare form of heart disease known as Reynaud's disease.

Side effects

The most serious undesirable action of the drug is orthostatic hypotension, a fall in blood pressure when the patient stands erect. Large doses can also cause rapid heartbeat. These effects probably arise from the nerve-blocking action of the compound. Certain others, including nasal congestion, dryness of the mouth, contraction of the pupils, drowsiness, sedation, loss of appetite, nausea and vomiting, are less frequent and are in part at least due to actions which are not understood.

Phenoxybenzamine and related agents are slow to act, and remain effective for three or four days. They ought not to be administered to a patient in whom a fall in blood pressure could be life threatening such as may be the case in the hardening of arteries in the brain, kidney damage, certain forms of heart disease or shock.

Chemistry and physiology

The haloalkylamines contain a halogen (chlorine, bromine, iodine and fluorine) bonded (see 'Biochemistry,') directly to an ethylamine:

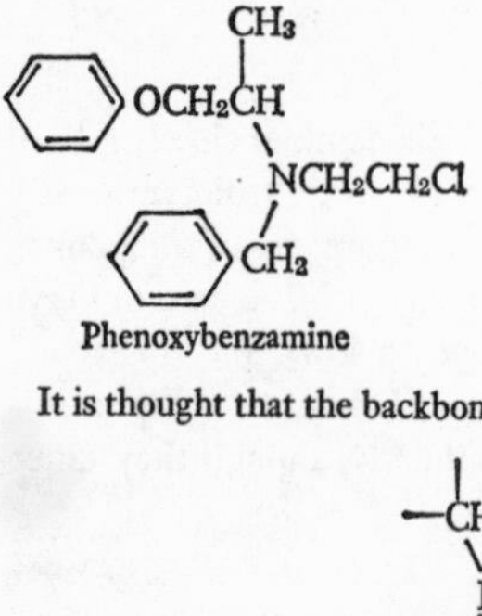

Cl = chlorine

NCH_2CH_2 = ethylamine

Phenoxybenzamine

It is thought that the backbone of the ethylamine chain forms a ring

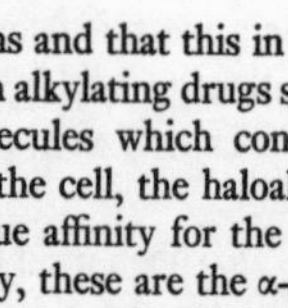

under biological conditions and that this in turn is broken to form an alkylating agent. Although alkylating drugs such as chlorambucil (q.v.) disrupt intracellular molecules which contain genetic information, thus damaging or killing the cell, the haloalkylamines appear to have a particular if not a unique affinity for the receptors for certain nervous impulses. Specifically, these are the α-adrenergic receptors, that is, the excitatory nerve or muscle cells of the sympathetic nervous system which normally respond to the chemical transmitter of nervous impulses, noradrenaline (see 'Adrenaline'). Because the chemical structure of these receptors is unknown, the molecular action of phenoxybenzamine is unclear.

Normally, α-receptors respond only to noradrenaline. (The halo-alkylamines may also block receptors for another chemical transmitter of nervous impulses, 5-hydroxytryptamine [5-HT, serotonin; see 'L-Dopa', 'Methyldopa' 'Phenelzine'].) This class of drugs alkylate the relevant receptors, thus inactivating them. The inactivation may involve bonds between the drug molecule and the receptor, though the fact that the inactivation gradually wears away suggests that the drug molecule is gradually broken down metabolically so that the α-receptors again become amenable to stimulation by noradrenaline.

The α-adrenergic receptor cells in smooth muscle (that which is not under voluntary control) include those in the peripheral blood vessels. The drug-induced blockade causes these muscles to relax, allowing blood pressure to fall. However, a fall in blood pressure sets up contradictory reflexes, especially in heart muscle, so that under certain conditions, the compound may induce a rise in blood pressure. The central nervous effects of the drugs and their effects on the gastrointestinal tract ('Side effects', above) are at least in part caused by actions other than the α-adrenergic blockade.

Poldine methylsulphate

(M. D. Mehta, 1955, U.K.) Trade names: Nacton, Nactisol. Administration: oral.

Classification

A synthetic substitute for the natural alkaloids (natural substances which are alkaline or basic as opposed to acid) of belladonna such as atropine (q.v.) developed in order to retain certain effects of these drugs on peripheral nerves while eliminating their undesirable actions on the central nervous system (CNS). Other agents which are chemically related, although their actions and therapeutic uses vary, include dibutoline, isopropamide, oxyphenonium, tricyclamol and valethamate.

Therapeutic uses

The major purpose of poldine methylsulphate is to control the pain of peptic or stomach ulcers. The agent reduces the secretions of gastric acid in the stomach, and thus helps to eliminate the pain caused by acid irritation of the raw sore in the stomach wall. The question whether a reduction in acid secretion and relief of pain also affords a better chance for the ulcer to heal has not been answered with certainty. The compound is, however, also useful in treatment of excess acid conditions, and it may be employed for relief of certain disorders related to the movement of the muscles in the intestinal walls.

Side effects

With normal doses, unwanted effects are rare and mild. They can include dryness of the mouth, slowness in urination, blurring of vision, rapid and erratic heartbeat, and even less frequently and with excessively high dosage, headache, belching and reduced sexual potency.

Chemistry and physiology

Like atropine, poldine is an anti-muscarinic compound; that is, one which blocks the action of part of the parasympathetic division of the autonomic nervous system (see 'Adrenaline'). This effect is thought to be achieved in part because the chemical binds to the receptor cells in smooth muscle of the eye, the intestine, the kidneys and other organs, and in part because it competes with acetylcholine (ACh), one of the chemical transmitters of nervous impulses between nerve cells in the CNS, between peripheral nerves, including those in parts of the parasympathetic system, and between certain nerves and the muscle cells they control. The molecular mechanism of action of the compound is not fully understood.

Poldine's usefulness derives from the fact that the secretion of gastric acid is in part at least controlled by parasympathetic nerves. The compound binds to receptors in cells of the stomach wall which are normally stimulated by ACh released from the nerve ends, thus interrupting signals from the brain which would otherwise increase gastric acid secretions. Such signals are reflex when there is food in the stomach, for example. Similarly, the drug is thought to enhance the motility or movement of the intestinal walls. In this action, however, the drug blocks impulses passing along nerves which normally stimulate muscles in the intestine to retain tone or rigidity. Certain diseases increase this rigidity to the point where food is moved along the gastrointestinal tract very slowly if at all.

The undesirable side effects of the drug probably occur because it also affects the CNS and the nerve ganglia, or nerve clusters outside the CNS, in a manner similar to atropine. That poldine exerts less action on the CNS than does atropine, and more on the peripheral nerves may be explained by several factors; e.g. its chemical structure, the structure of the receptor molecule and the amount of each drug which it is necessary to administer in order to obtain the desired therapeutic results.

Pralidoxime

(Wilson and Ginsberg, 1955, U.S., and Childs, *et al.*, 1955, U.K.) Trade name: U.S. Protopam. Not available commercially in U.K. Administration: injection.

Classification
One of the hundreds of compounds affecting the transmission of nerve impulses by altering one of the relevant natural substances involved in the process of carrying a message between one nerve cell and the next in line, or between a nerve and the muscle which it regulates. ('Chemistry and physiology', below. This entry should be read in conjunction with entries on 'Atropine' and 'Neostigmine'.) The agent was synthesized in a search for antidotes to poisoning by insecticides such as parathion and malathion, and by organophosphorous 'nerve gases'. Related compounds include diacetylmonoxime (DAM) and monoisonitrosoacetone (MINA).

Therapeutic uses
The major importance of pralidoxime is as an antidote for accidental poisoning by certain insecticides, and as treatment for excessive dosage with neostigmine (q.v.) when this drug is being used to control myasthenia gravis, and acute weakening of the muscles in the arms, legs and face. Pralidoxime is usually given with atropine (q.v.). The drug may also be used to prevent poisoning among workers employed in the manufacture of insecticides.

Side effects
These may include dizziness, vision disturbances, nausea, an erratic increase in heart rate, headache, drowsiness, rapid deep breathing and muscular weakness.

Chemistry and physiology

Pralidoxime is an anti-anti-cholinesterase; that is, it antagonizes compounds such as neostigmine which inhibit cholinesterase (AChE). AChE is an intercellular enzyme, one formed within cells but active in the spaces between them. It rapidly catalyses the breakdown of acetylcholine (ACh), the substance which transmits nervous impulses between nerves in the parasympathetic division of the autonomic nervous system (see 'Adrenaline'), and between nerves and muscles in parts of the autonomic nervous system as well as the voluntary network. Under certain conditions, (e.g. glaucoma), it is desirable to reduce or stop normal transmission. For this purpose a drug such as atropine may be employed because it blocks ACh. However, under other conditions, including myasthenia gravis, it is necessary to enhance transmission by inhibiting the enzyme, AChE, which normally destroys ACh. But too much ACh can cause tetany, a rigidity of the muscles; if tetany occurs, an antidote is required to unblock the catabolic enzyme. This is the role of pralidoxime.

The drug works because it tends to combine with a molecule of the compound which is inhibiting AChE, if the inhibitory drug is an organophosphorous compound; that is, one containing the structure:

$$H_7C_3O \diagdown \diagup OC_3H_7 \\ P-O^- \\ \| \\ R$$

P = phosphorus
R = a positively charged ion (q.v.)
O⁻ = a negatively charged oxygen ion

When the drug combines with this molecule, it alters the charges on the atoms so that the molecule is released from its bond to AChE. The latter is then again available to catalyse the breakdown of ACh.

Progesterone

(Synthesized by Butenandt, *et al.*, 1934, Ger.) Trade names: (microcrystalline form): Micryston progesterone. Administration: oral ('Oral contraceptives', below), injection.

Classification

The main natural progestin (see 'Hormone'), originally isolated from sows and normally present in the female mainly in the second half of the menstrual cycle and during pregnancy. Pure progesterone is almost inactive taken by mouth, and has to be given by injection, even following which its duration of action is very short. Thus the natural compound is rarely used and has largely been replaced either by long-acting esters (see 'Biochemistry') such as hydroxyprogesterone caproate, or by related compounds such as medroxyprogesterone acetate, chlormadinone acetate or norethisterone, which are active when given orally. Other related compounds are ethisterone, dimethisterone, norethynodrel, lynoestrenol, norgestrel, ethynodiol diacetate and megestrol acetate.

Therapeutic uses
Without doubt the widest use of these compounds today is in oral contraceptives. However, they are also used in certain gynaecological conditions, and in the field of cancer therapy both within and outside the genital tract.

One of the most controversial uses of progestins is in the treatment of threatened or habitual abortion. The condition is thought to occur because of a postulated deficiency of progesterone production by either the corpus luteum (see 'Hormones') or the placenta, particularly around the time of pregnancy when the main source of supply of this compound changes from the former to the latter. Considerable success with progestins was described as long as thirty years ago, but unfortunately, these early studies have not been well confirmed, a situation for which a number of possible explanations may be suggested. For example, it is often thought that if several abortions have occurred, the next pregnancy will almost certainly follow suit – an assumption for which there is little statistical evidence – and it is not surprising therefore that progestin treatment in such cases may often be followed by a normal birth at full term, a result which would have occurred even without the treatment. In addition there is evidence that abortion often occurs because of an early malformed foetus; if progestin therapy was really successful one would expect its application to be followed by a higher than normal incidence of abnormal infants, which is not the case. Thus the case for progestin therapy in habitual abortion must remain at best 'Not proven', although it is certainly possible that, by virtue of their sedative effect, progestins may help to tide over the nervous woman through a critical stage of her pregnancy during which she might otherwise abort for nervous or emotional reasons.

The compounds may be used for diagnosis of pregnancy after a missed period, although such use is now falling into disrepute. In the female menstruation occurs as a result of withdrawal of hormonal support from a well-developed uterine lining (endometrium). In pregnancy, however, such withdrawal does not occur and menstruation does not take place.

Decreased ovarian function, or lack of ovulation with

consequent lack of progesterone production from the corpus luteum, may also cause missed menstruation. To differentiate between these conditions (i.e. pregnancy or altered ovarian function), oestrogen (see 'Oestradiol')–progestin combinations may be given for a few days and then withdrawn. If the patient is pregnant, no bleeding will normally occur because of the presence of endogenous (natural) hormonal support; if she is not pregnant, hormone-withdrawal bleeding may be expected.

Progesterone alone may sometimes be used in women who continually miss periods (amenorrhoea) to demonstrate whether or not the ovary is at all active. In women with prolonged, heavy or irregular periods too, regularization of the cycle with decrease in the amount and frequency of the periods can be achieved, although many doctors now prefer to use oestrogen/progestin combinations similar to those in oral contraceptives for this purpose. Similarly dysmenorrhoea (painful periods) and endometriosis (an unusual condition in which little bits of endometrium become located in sites outside the uterus and give rise to bleeding cysts, pain and tenderness) which used to be treated with progestins alone are now frequently attended to with preparations containing oestrogen also.

Occasionally the lining of the womb may undergo changes which lead to cancer, cells from which may break off into the bloodstream and land in other organs (for example, the lungs), there giving rise to secondary deposits called metastases. Because of its effect in altering the growth of endometrial cells, the synthethic progestogens are extremely effective in controlling these growths and, indeed, in decreasing their size.

In breast cancer, too, the use of progestogens alone can bring about some very good results, although here the mechanism of action (unless it be to oppose the action of oestrogen on which many of these tumours appear to depend) is less certain. There is a possibility that these tumours may also require prolactin (see 'Hormones') for their growth, and that the production of this substance from the pituitary may be inhibited by progestogens. However, in the absence of a good assay method for prolactin, this suggestion must remain uncertain.

Recently certain progesterone derivatives have been discovered to have the rather novel action of opposing the effects of the male hormones (see 'Testosterone') in the body; in other words, they are anti-androgenic. This discovery opened the way for the development of a number of new therapeutic entities in such fields as the control of acne, hair growth and baldness, the control of sexual offenders, the amelioration of the overgrowth of the prostate gland which affects almost one man out of every two over the age of fifty, and a possible control for cancer of the same gland which may lack the risks of thrombosis (blood clots) attributed to the only other effective form of therapy in this condition currently available – namely, oestrogens.

Side effects

Progesterone itself (and indeed most of the synthetic compounds) is remarkably free of side effects. Certain well-recognized symptoms which appear particularly in the female towards the latter part of her menstrual cycle may be ascribed to a dominance of progesterone in her hormonal balance, however, and include temporary weight gain (due to anabolic action – see 'Metabolism'), premenstrual tension, possibly depression and leg cramps (although the evidence on these is confused, to say the least) and acne. An androgenic (see 'Hormone') effect of certain of the synthetic compounds, has been alleged, but is not well proven.

Chemistry and physiology

The formula of progesterone, of the injectable compound hydroxyprogesterone caproate, and of two examples of the main types of orally active progestins, are given below. It is noticeable that the injectable preparation is basically an ester (see 'Biochemistry') of progesterone in which a long side chain is added to prolong the activity of the compound, which is otherwise natural progesterone. In the case of the orally active compounds, however, molecular alterations have been made which divide them into two main types: the 17-acetoxy compounds, of which chlormadinone acetate is an example, and the 19-nor compounds, of which norethisterone is an example.

Basically all of the progestogens have similar physiological activities, although the degree to which they separately exhibit progestogenicity, anti-oestrogenicity, anti-androgenicity and even occasionally oestrogenicity and androgenicity is variable. In one particularly effective means of assessing activity the following relative progestogenic potencies have been observed with some of the more commonly used compounds.

Relative Progestogenic Potency	
Norethisterone	1·0
Megestrol	1·5
Norethisterone acetate	2·0
Ethynodiol diacetate	15·0
Norgestrel	30·0

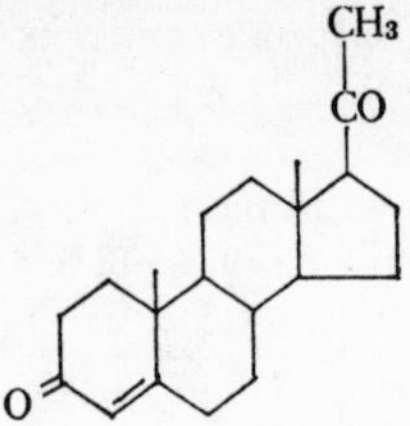

Progesterone

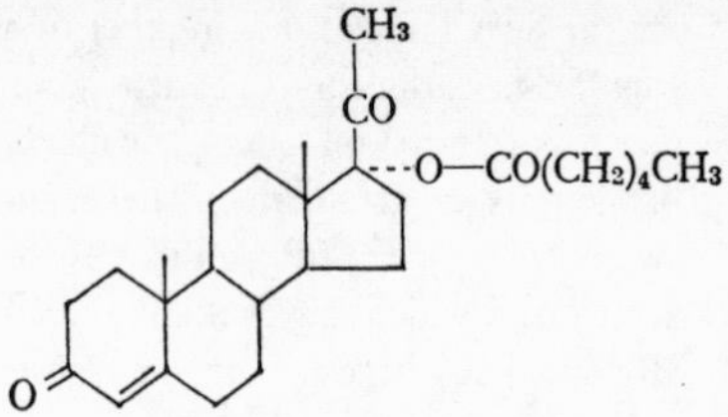

Hydroxyprogesterone caproate

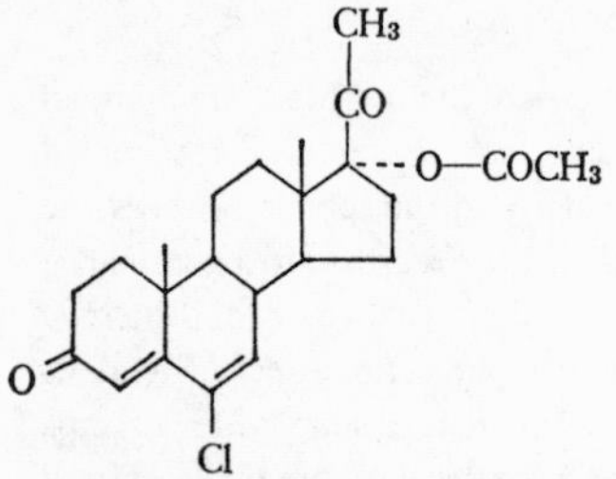

Chlormadinone acetate

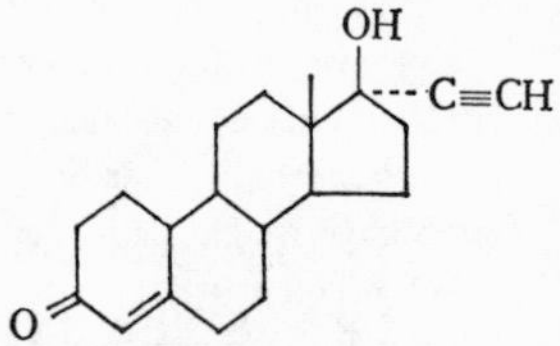

Norethisterone

Potencies of these compounds vary widely in this test, and it is this variation, in combination with the variability in their other pharmacological activities, which give to the different progestogens their distinctive advantages in differing situations.

The effect of progesterone in inhibiting luteinizing hormone release from the pituitary (see 'Hormones') presumably imparts to certain of the synthetic compounds their efficacy in bringing about the inhibition of ovulation (although effects on follicle-stimulating hormone levels may also be involved). This property too varies widely from one compound to another; for example, chlormadinone acetate in doses of up to 0·5 mg daily may not inhibit ovulation while norethisterone in half that dose is extremely effective.

Progesterone is produced principally during the second half of the menstrual cycle from the corpus luteum in the ovary. Its main peripheral effect is on the endometrium where it converts the rapidly growing and proliferating cells into secretory ones which produce the fluid-containing nutriment necessary for the development of the fertilized ovum. In addition progesterone brings about a further thickening of the endometrium to prepare it for implantation. In the latest part of the menstrual cycle it causes changes in the cells of the endometrium called decidualization, which may protect the womb from overactive invasion by the implanting embryo. At the level of the cervix (the neck of the womb), progesterone appears to affect the mucus plug to make it less receptive to sperm penetration. It is possible that the 'mini-pill' oral contraceptives which do not contain oestrogen and may not inhibit ovulation achieve their antifertility effect in this manner.

Progestogens also have a thermogenic effect, that is, they bring about a rise in the body temperature. In the normally cycling woman the oral temperature taken in the morning before rising, the basal body temperature, shows a rise of about 1° F at the time of ovulation which persists thereafter until near the end of the cycle. This is generally thought to be due to the production of progesterone, and can be demonstrated by giving progestogens to men. It is often used with rather misguided zeal as a method of birth control too, with resulting pregnancy rates which can be up to thirty-five per cent or more!

Towards the end of the menstrual cycle it is not uncommon for women to complain of a feeling of tenderness, and even of nodularity, in their breasts. This is almost certainly an effect of progesterone, acting in concert with oestrogen, on the secretory tissue of the breast, and represents in a minor form the changes which appear more grossly during pregnancy, and which prepare the breast for milk production after parturition. Immediately after childbirth the high levels of circulating oestrogens and progesterone diminish sharply, and this may precipitate lactation, either directly, or indirectly through removal of an inhibition of pituitary hormone production necessary for the process.

Perhaps the most important physiological role for progesterone is in the maintenance of pregnancy. In the first three months of pregnancy the steroid is produced from the corpus luteum, but thereafter the placenta takes over this role, and ever larger amounts are produced right up to the time of childbirth. That the steroid is required for maintenance is demonstrated by the occurrence of abortion if the ovary, and corpus luteum therein, is removed before the third month.

The action of progesterone at the cellular level has not been clearly elucidated for all tissues upon which it acts. Unlike oestrogen it does not appear to be specifically localized to sensitive tissues in the body, although it can stimulate ribonucleic acid (RNA) synthesis in isolated nuclei of cells in certain receptive tissues, presumably by increasing RNA-polymerase activity (see 'Actinomycin D'). In the rat uterus, also, it has been shown to enhance the uptake of radioactive oestrogen by the endometrial cell nuclei, and the possibility that it acts, in that site at least, in co-operation with oestrogen cannot be excluded.

Oral contraceptives

Three generations of oral contraceptives have appeared. Of these the first, the combined oral contraceptive in which both oestrogen and progestogen are given together from day 5 to day 20 or 21 of the cycle, followed by a seven-day gap, is still by far the most popular. The second, the sequential preparations in which oestrogen alone is given for the first fourteen days followed by seven days of oestrogen/progestogen combination, again with a seven-day gap, are claimed to be more similar to natural physiological sequences, but it has largely come to grief (at least in the United Kingdom) on the grounds of lower efficacy in preventing pregnancy. Both of these types of preparation depend on inhibition of ovulation for their mechanism of action although combined preparations containing the anti-oestrogenic steroid, norethisterone, or its derivatives may also offer two further means of protection by making the endometrium hostile to implantation, and by making the cervical mucus plug impenetrable to sperm. The inhibition of ovulation is produced by operation of the feedback mechanism by exogenously administered steroids in the preparations, and inhibition of production of pituitary hormones necessary for follicular development and/or ovulation.

Unlike the first two generations of oral contraceptives the third probably depends, for its contraceptive efficacy, mainly on the cervical mucus effect, preventing entry of spermatozoa into the uterus, although the possibility that interference with the preparation of the sperm for fertilization (capacitation), which normally occurs in the uterus, has not been excluded. Inhibition of ovulation appears to be variable with different preparations of this type. Unfortunately the first of these 'mini-pill' preparations to be made available, chlormadinone acetate alone, has had to be withdrawn from the market due to the appearance of breast nodules in dogs treated with large doses of the drug. However, it is still quite possible that the effects of steroids on dogs are irrelevant to their effects on women. Alternatively, other 'mini-pills' free from this effect may become available.

Oral contraceptives, with the exception of the progestogen-only 'mini-pills', all contain mixtures of oestrogens (either ethinyl-oestradiol or mestranol) and various progestogens. Despite claims to the contrary, it is doubtful whether any one preparation, except in terms of steroid quantity administered, presents significant therapeutic advantages over any other. However, recently the Scowen (formerly Dunlop) Committee on Drug Safety has indicated that preparations containing more that 50 μg of oestrogen show statistically a higher risk of thrombosis than preparations containing less oestrogen. It would seem logical therefore to use preparations which offer, both in terms of steroid weight and of potency, the lowest quantity of oestrogen compatible with maximum contraceptive efficacy.

The uses of oral contraceptives are considerable. Quite apart from their widespread self-administration for conception control, they are utilized for treatment of dysmenorrhoea, cycle irregularity, menopausal upsets, excessive menstrual bleeding and, in increased dosage, for endometriosis. In all of these conditions they are effective, as indeed they are in the prevention of pregnancy.

True side effects of oral contraceptives are rare. The very few which can be probably laid at the door of these preparations are nausea, occasional vomiting, headache and discomfort in the breasts, all of which may be expected to disappear after the first two or three cycles. Numerous other complaints have been associated with 'The Pill', but it is likely that these represent 'scapegoat' reactions by women who still believe, even if only subconsciously, that sex is something to be endured rather than enjoyed. A statistical adverse reaction to oral contraceptives which has been observed is the occurrence of thrombosis, which may be fatal, in a very small number of women on oestrogen-containing pills. The risk is around 3 per 100,000 women on 'The Pill'; and if they had become pregnant, a larger number would have died due to complications of pregnancy. Had *all 100,000* decided to use mechanical means of contraception even more would have died due to pregnancy complications, as the failure rate of all of these methods is fairly high. Indeed, the risk of being killed crossing the road (one which we tend to accept) is of the order of 6 per 100,000, and the risk of 'The Pill' is about equivalent to that of smoking seven cigarettes *a month*.

Does 'The Pill' cause cancer? This question has been asked repeatedly and still remains one of the major 'back of the mind' worries for the woman on 'The Pill'. Certainly some of the steroids in 'The Pill' if given to animals in enormous doses (up to two hundred times the human dose) over periods corresponding to more than half the life-span of a woman may cause cancer in these animals. But there is no evidence to indicate that these studies have any relevance to human beings, and, indeed, considerable evidence that they do not. As regards breast cancer, in particular, a recent report has suggested that use of 'The Pill' may possibly protect against development of this disease, and similar suggestions regarding pre-cancerous changes in the cervix have been made. Certainly, in neither case has the use of 'The

Pill' over relatively long periods been associated with an increased occurrence of the condition.

Indeed, it is unfortunate that over-reaction to alleged side effects is threatening to inhibit their use in an already over-crowded world. Yet agitation against oral contraceptives amounts to a campaign for their removal from the market. Even if a perfect preparation were available to enter clinical trials now, it would take at least ten years before drug-regulatory authorities and less authoritative critics of 'The Pill' were satisfied and the new compounds generally available. Such is the rate of the population explosion, by that time it would be too late!

All oral contraceptives now on the market are designed for use by women. Work is also going forward on a 'pill' for men, an oral contraceptive that would make men temporarily infertile while not impairing potency or inducing permanent sterility. One compound, trimethylphosphate (TMP), has kept rats infertile for a year after dosage at two-weekly intervals. Fertility returned when the animals were taken off TMP, and few unwanted side effects have been noted. Tests of such compounds on humans remain to be undertaken.

Propranolol

(Black, *et al.*, 1964, U.K.) Trade name: Inderal. Administration: oral, or by intravenous injection.

Classification

Synthesized in the course of a planned search for a drug with selective action on certain muscles, particularly heart muscle, which receive nervous impulses from a part of the sympathetic division of the autonomic nervous system ('Chemistry and physiology', below; see also 'Adrenaline'). Propranolol is chemically similar to pronethalol and dichloroisoproterenol, both of which it has superseded in clinical practice.

Therapeutic uses

The compound is used principally for treatment of certain forms of heart disease. It is particularly effective in preventing angina pectoris, an acute and painful 'heart attack' which occurs when heart muscle suffers a shortage of oxygen and other nutrients.

Because the drug is thought to reduce heart-muscle requirements for oxygen, it is also useful for the treatment of heart attacks caused by blockages in blood vessels feeding heart muscle (myocardial infarction). Disturbances in heartbeat rhythms (arrhythmias), especially those which cannot be controlled or are caused by digitalis, may respond well to propranolol.

Under some circumstances, the agent may reduce high blood pressure (hypertension), though the effect requires several days of drug administration to appear. When propranolol is used with a drug such as phenoxybenzamine (q.v.), however, it will promptly control hypertension caused by a tumour of the adrenal gland called phaeochromocytoma.

There is some evidence that the compound controls the tremor of Parkinson's disease, and that it can reduce the rapid heartbeat caused by an overactive thyroid gland.

Side effects

These are relatively rare, but may include nausea, vomiting, diarrhoea, insomnia, lassitude and unsteadiness. Skin rashes, hallucinations and paresthesia have occurred even less often after use of the drug.

If it is administered during anaesthesia, it can cause dangerous slowing of heart rate though this can be corrected with atropine (q.v.). The agent tends to cause constriction of bronchial tubes and air passages in the lungs, and should be employed with great care for patients with asthma, bronchitis or emphysema.

Chemistry and physiology

At the molecular level, propranolol is thought to act by altering the activity of an enzyme, adenyl cyclase, in a manner that leads to lower levels of an intracellular substance called cyclic AMP (see 'Hormone', p. 122).

The muscle cells which are relevant to this effect contain molecular sites known as beta-adrenergic (literally: energized by adrenaline, q.v.) receptors. These sites normally respond chemically, when they are met by molecules of noradrenaline, the substance which transmits nerve impulses between nerve ends and between nerve ends and muscle cells in the sympathetic and parts of the parasympathetic divisions of the autonomic nervous system. At least two types of adrenergic receptors are believed to exist: α-receptors are usually excitatory; that is, they cause muscles in the cells of which they occur to contract. Beta-receptors, on the other hand, are usually inhibitory, or relaxing. Two types of receptors have been identified: β_1 receptors, as found in the heart, and β_2 receptors, as found in the bronchi. This classification is based on their differential response to β-blockers such as propranolol and to drugs that stimulate β-receptors (see below), and may explain the apparent contradictory behaviour of heart muscle where cells contain β-receptors, but are excitatory. Thus, propranolol, a beta-blocking agent, tends to slow heartbeat and to control arrhythmias. Its antihypertensive action probably stems in the main from the relaxation induced in muscles which constrict certain peripheral blood vessels. The reason for its reported anti-parkinsonian action is unclear, but any drug which affects the transmission of nervous impulses may have a variety of actions on the brain as well as the peripheral nerves. Because this class of compound is relatively new, these complex relationships are by no means well understood.

The expansion of knowledge about β-adrenergic receptors founded in part on experiment with blocking agents such as propranolol has, however, led to the development of improved beta-adrenergic stimulants such as isoprenaline (β_1 stimulant) and salbutamol (β_2 stimulant). Early β-blockers, because of relatively non-specific action on β_1 receptors, could be dangerous when given to asthmatics, but recent work has led to development of new compounds such as practolol which are more specific for β_1 receptors, and less likely to cause bronchoconstriction in the asthmatic patient.

Prostaglandin

One of a class of natural substances found in all human tissues and all animal species so far investigated. The word was coined by U. S. von Euler, a Swedish scientist; in 1935, he identified a factor in seminal fluid and prostate gland extracts that caused certain muscles such as those in the uterus and intestine to contract.

The original prostaglandin has since been shown to contain at least thirteen different compounds, though all of them are closely related chemically and have very similar molecular structures. All of them appear to be formed from fat-like substances in the body.

Like most hormones (q.v.), but unlike enzymes (q.v.), the prostaglandin molecules are small and relatively simple. Again, like hormones, these substances drastically modify cellular behaviour. They appear to be transported in blood and lymphatic fluid, and to act in part at least at distances from their sites of biosynthesis. On the other hand, their apparent ubiquity and their relatively constant presence as well as evidence that they act in the tissues where they are formed, require that they be looked upon as local hormones (see 'Hormone', final section of entry) if indeed the word is applicable to them at all.

The public became aware of prostaglandins in 1970 as a result of clinical trials of two of them in particular, PGE_2 and $PGF_{2\alpha}$ (PG = prostaglandin; E and F are two of the four major subgroups of chemicals, the others being identified as A and B; the number 2 and the letter α (alpha) refer to certain aspects of molecular configuration). $PGF_{2\alpha}$ and PGE_2 as well as $FT_{1\alpha}$ and E_1 have been used for some time to induce natural childbirth at normal term. In January 1970 an article in *The Lancet* described the induction of abortions in the ninth to the twenty-second week in fourteen out of fifteen cases by the slow injection of $PGF_{2\alpha}$. No serious side effects were observed though there was some diarrhoea and vomiting. PGE_2 was subsequently used in smaller amounts with similar successful results and without diarrhoea.

Several pharmaceutical houses have begun intensive research, one of the major objectives of which is production of an abortifacient pill, that is, an abortion inducer that could, for example, be taken once a month at the time of normal menstruation so that if the woman is pregnant, she will abort, whereas if she is not, she will have her normal period. The difficulties are chiefly two, apart from religious or moral considerations: (1) natural prostaglandins are destroyed by digestive juices so that either it will be necessary to synthesize an artificial agent that will resist destruction until it can be absorbed into the bloodstream, or another method of administration will have to be found. At least one house, working along the latter line, has developed a plastic disc that can be inserted without surgery directly into the uterus, where it will remain for periods of a year or more. (2) Any new drug, even a natural substance, may have side effects that can be identified only after long and varied trials. Indeed, the natural substances now appear to cause serious side effects that make them unsuitable for the regulation of fertility, and there is an intensive search for synthetic agents with similar abortifacient effects which are less toxic.

In the seminal vesicles and prostate, one or more prostaglandins are thought to be responsible for the rapid contractions that cause ejaculation. In the uterus, they may be responsible in part for the contractions of childbirth, and in the intestine, for normal peristalsis. Yet prostaglandins do not cause contraction in all smooth muscle, the tissues in the uterus and intestine under involuntary control as opposed to the striated muscles of the arms and legs that are under voluntary control. (Heart muscle is considered to be a third type of muscular tissue; see 'Digitalis'.)

These substances have striking though often contradictory effects, moreover, in the brain and spinal cord, the lungs, kidneys and the blood vessels. They are thought to be one factor in the 'cascade' that leads to inflammation (see 'Aspirin'), and they and their metabolites (see 'Metabolism') appear to be involved in the spasms characteristic of asthma. The prostaglandins also play a role in the functioning of the iris in the eye. Other biological effects have been reported in a mass of experimental data involving at least ten genera.

Not surprisingly, their molecular mechanism of action is also unclear. They may antagonize certain intracellular enzymes, or they may alter the properties of cellular membranes or of the movement of ions (q.v.), especially calcium ions, within cells. Experimental evidence suggests that like many substances including many drugs, the prostaglandin molecules attach to specific 'receptor' molecules on or in cells in order to exert their effects, but the nature of such receptors is unknown.

One of the synthetic prostaglandins is now available for hospital use only, in obstetrics.

Streptomycin

(Schatz, Waksman and Bugie, 1944, U.S.) Trade names: Strepolin, Strepaquaine. Administration: injection, orally for intestinal diseases; eye and ear drops.

Classification

The second antibiotic (q.v.) to be developed (after penicillin; q.v.), streptomycin was discovered as the result of an intensive and well-planned research programme to screen potentially useful organisms. The programme affords an example of cooperation between a government agency, the National Research Council of the United States which organized it and the pharmaceutical companies which financed it.

Streptomycin is produced by *Streptomyces griseus* and certain other bacteria. Like penicillin, it is a narrow-spectrum antibiotic because the range of organisms which it either kills or inhibits is limited. Unlike penicillin, however, this agent attacks some Gram-negative as well as Gram-positive bacteria (see 'Antibiotic').

Therapeutic uses

Streptomycin is most frequently employed in the treatment and cure of tuberculosis. The drug itself probably does not kill all of the causative bacteria, but reduces the population sufficiently so that the natural immunological defences of the body can dispose of the remainder. In order to delay the development of bacterial resistance ('Chemistry and physiology', below), streptomycin is usually given with other anti-tuberculosis drugs such as isoniazid (q.v.), sodium aminosalicylate, ethionamide and pyrazinamide. Those forms of the disease against which the antibiotic is most effective include tuberculous meningitis, miliary or disseminated tuberculosis, pulmonary tuberculosis in the early stages or when it is progressing rapidly, and, in many cases, tuberculosis of the mouth, tongue, throat, windpipe, bronchial tubes and the genito-urinary tract.

With penicillin, streptomycin is used against infections of heart muscle caused by certain streptococcal bacteria, and for peritonitis caused by mixed streptococcal and clostridial (genus: *Clostridium*) infections.

Plague is effectively treated with the drug, as are tularaemia (in combination with a sulphonamide, q.v.) and brucellosis (in combination with tetracycline, q.v.). Infections of the urinary tract caused by some bacteria may also be eliminated by the agent. Under certain circumstances, gonorrhoea, a form of pneumonia and bacillary dysentery respond well to it.

Side effects

Few undesirable reactions occur when the drug is administered orally, possibly because it is poorly absorbed through the intestine. It must usually be injected for treatment of systemic diseases or those centred outside the intestinal tract. Minor signs of slight poisoning by streptomycin may include pricking sensations or numbness around the mouth, vertigo, headache and lassitude as well as pain and irritation at the site of injection.

In rare cases, after massive injections into the abdomen, respiratory arrest can occur. If large doses are given orally, especially in combination with other antibiotics, some bacteria normally occurring in the intestine will be destroyed. Those which remain may multiply rapidly leading to a rare condition called super-infection. This can be fatal.

Allergy-like hypersensitivity reactions occur more often, and can also be serious. They may include fever, skin disorders and enlargement of the lymph glands. Workmen employed in manufacture of the drug and nurses and pharmacists who handle it can also develop skin rashes.

Streptomycin in large and continuous doses can damage the inner ear, particularly the organs responsible for balance, and the nerves leading from the ear to the hearing centre in the brain. Permanent vertigo or deafness can result. This unfortunate effect is less frequent if the patient is under the age of forty.

Liver and kidney damage may also result from large doses of the agent. It should be given to patients with liver and kidney diseases only with the greatest care, and never to those with diseases of the ear.

Chemistry and physiology

Streptomycin is a complex molecule composed of a sugar, a sugar-amine combination and a moiety called streptidine. Its mechanism of action is uncertain, but the drug probably interferes with bacterial synthesis of protein. It appears to bind to intracellular organelles called ribosomes. These are little machines for the manufacture of protein molecules common to all cells. The ribosome receives instructions from the gene-bearing deoxyribonucleic acid (DNA) molecule in the form of a molecule of messenger ribonucleic acid (m-RNA) which has been patterned on the DNA template. The m-RNA attaches to a ribosome where it selects other molecules of transfer RNA (t-RNA) which carry appropriate amino acids, and lines them up in the proper order to produce the protein specified by that m-RNA. The ribosome connects the amino acids together by means of peptide bonds (see 'Biochemistry'). Streptomycin is thought to interfere at the stage where the t-RNA is bound to the m-RNA, thus disrupting the sequence of protein assemblage. It is unclear whether this drug action also applies to mammalian cells, and if it does, whether the resultant cell damage causes any of the unwanted side effects.

Some bacteria can actually grow on low concentrations of streptomycin, but the vast majority are either sensitive to the drug, or resistant. The difference is of course inherited, and apparently stems from differences in the structure of ribosomes as between the two types, but resistance can appear very rapidly in previously sensitive families of bacteria. This phenomenon is obviously a serious clinical problem. It may be caused by mutation, by the selective survival of resistant strains within the sensitive family or by some direct effect of the drug on the bacterium. To delay the appearance of resistant strains, streptomycin may be administered with sulphonamides or other drugs, though not with other antibiotics ('Therapeutic uses' and 'Side effects', above).

Sulphonamide. U.S.: Sulfonamide

One of a class of synthetic anti-bacterial drugs derived from sulphanilamide, the first in the series. Originally synthesized in 1908 (Gelmo, Ger.) in the investigation of new dyes for cloth, the antibacterial potency of sulphanilamide and related compounds was recognized as early as 1917. It was not until Domagk (Ger.) discovered the therapeutic usefulness of a new dye, prontosil, in 1932, however, that the drug was tested clinically. It remained for a group of French scientists, Nitti, Bovet and the Trefouëls, to demonstrate three years later that the active chemical in prontosil is sulphanilamide.

Chemical variations on the basic molecule, with differing pharmacological properties, appeared swiftly. Over 5,400 have been investigated, but fewer than twenty continue in active clinical use. Among the most important of these are sulphadiazine, with probably the highest anti-bacterial potency of any drug in the class, sulphamerazine, succinylsulphathiazole and phthalylsulphathiazole, sulphacetamide and sulphisoxazole, sulphamethoxypyridazine and sulphadimethoxine.

On a dose basis, the antibiotics (q.v.) are much more potent than the sulphonamides. This and certain other disadvantages have diminished the role of the latter in clinical practice. Treatment with both an antibiotic and a sulphonamide is customary in some forms of meningitis (streptomycin (q.v.), chloramphenicol or penicillin (q.v.) with sulphadiazine or sulphisoxazole), and in a lung infection caused by an agent, *Nocardia asteroides*, which can lead to tuberculosis (tetracycline (q.v.) or streptomycin with sulphadiazine). Sulphonamides are combined with other drugs for treatment of infections caused by bacteria called *Toxoplasma* (pyrimethamine; see 'Quinacrine'. In the case of eye infections caused by these agents, the sulphonamide is combined with a corticosteroid; see 'Hormone').

A new drug (1968; trade name: Septrin) combines a sulphonamide, sulphamethoxazole, with a non-sulphonamide drug, trimethoprim, which is also a folic acid inhibitor (see below) for the treatment of acute bronchitis and certain urinary tract infections. However, in acute infections of the urinary tract, sulphamethoxypyridazine or sulphadimethoxine may be used as drugs of first choice. Similarly, sulphadiazine, sulphisoxazole or sulpha combinations (see below) may be preferred for control and prevention of bacillary dysentery, an acute and often fatal disease, although resistant causative bacteria are known to exist. Sulphadiazine and sulphisoxazole are drugs of first choice for treatment and prevention of meningitis caused by meningococcus, and for certain diseases of the eye, including trachoma (see also rifampicin, under 'Antibiotic').

Sulphonamides are classified under three headings on the basis of the rapidity with which they are absorbed through the intestinal wall, and excreted, principally via the kidneys. Agents absorbed and excreted rapidly include sulphadiazine and sulphisoxazole, as well as the sulpha combinations (see below). Sulphamethoxypyridazine and sulphadimethoxine are absorbed rapidly and excreted slowly. They are, therefore, more useful for treatment of chronic illnesses or for prophylaxis (the prevention of infection). Succinylsulphathiazole and phthalylsulphathiazole are absorbed very poorly from the intestine and are used to reduce bacterial populations in the intestinal tract, particularly in the large intestine and colon, before surgery on these organs.

The sulphonamides are derivatives of a simple molecule which is related to an essential segment, para-aminobenzoic acid (PABA), of folic acid, a vitamin (q.v.) necessary among other things for the proper functioning of blood-element-forming cells in the bone marrow.

Sulphanilamide
(para-aminobenzene-
sulphonamide) H_2N—⬡—SO_2NH_2

PABA H_2N—⬡—$COOH$

Although bacteria do not of course contain anything resembling blood, folic acid is essential as a prosthetic group in enzymes (q.v.) common to most life forms. Many Gram-positive and Gram-negative bacteria (see 'Antibiotic') cannot incorporate pre-formed folic acid, but must synthesize their own supplies from constituent chemicals, including PABA. Because of the similarity in molecular structure, sulphonamides compete with PABA in the biosynthetic process, and prevent formation of folic acid. Bacterial cells stop growing normally and eventually die. However, the sulphonamides are considered to be bacterio-static rather than bactericidal drugs because, like many anti-biotics, they slow the development of bacterial populations and permit the body's natural immune-defence mechanisms (see discussion under 'Azathioprine') to immobilize and destroy the infective agents.

Although their most frequent mechanism of action is probably the inhibition of bacterial folic acid formation, the sulphon-amides can interfere with other metabolic processes. Thus, their selective attack on bacteria occurs because mammalian cells cannot synthesize folic acid, but must ingest the vitamin pre-formed, but their serious side effects appear to arise because of other less well understood actions which can alter the behaviour of mammalian cells as well as that of bacteria.

As with antibiotics, resistance to sulphonamide therapy is a phenomenon of the bacteria, not of the patient. That is, in-fective agents which have given way to treatment by these drugs slowly cease to respond.

It is thought that this resistance develops because some in-dividuals in any bacterial population are genetically capable of synthesizing enough PABA to antagonize the drug. As the bacteria unable to perform this synthesis die off, the resistant strain takes over. However, other resistance mechanisms may also be operating.

It is to overcome drug resistance that combination therapy with antibiotics and other agents is used. Sulphonamide mix-tures, on the other hand, are used to prevent certain side effects which are fairly common, particularly damage to the kidney and urinary tract from crystals of the metabolized drug (see 'Metabolism') often formed in the urine. The sulphonamide combinations include sulphadiazine with sulphamerazine or sulphacetamide, and possibly a third constituent, usually sulpha-methazine. These combinations are both absorbed and excreted fairly rapidly (see above), but the use of two or three drugs in the same solution does not significantly increase the plasma level of the agent. Rather the rationale behind the use of such mixtures arises from the fact that many substances can coexist in solution without interfering with their respective solubility. Thus, more sulphonamide can appear in the urine with less chance that it will precipitate out into crystals.

Probably the least toxic sulphonamide is sulphisoxazole; about 0·1 per cent of patients given the agent suffer serious untoward effects. The average for all drugs of the class is about 5 per cent. Although they are not common, the most serious side effects are blood disorders. These and the somewhat more frequent damage to the kidneys and urinary tract can of course be fatal. The most serious blood disorder, destruction of red blood cells, occurs more frequently in black than in white patients, and in children than in adults. It is thought that the disturbance occurs in patients whose red blood cells are deficient in an enzyme (q.v.), glucose-6-phosphate dehydrogenase, which is essential for the metabolism (q.v.) of carbohydrates (see 'Biochemistry').

However, the destruction of red blood cells may also occur because of an allergic-type reaction to the drugs. Skin eruptions, illnesses called serum sickness and drug fever, and hepatitis may also be caused by adverse responses of natural body defences to the agents. Because these side effects are unpredictable, and because when they occur the patient cannot in most cases be treated again with sulphonamides, their indiscriminate use is very unwise. This stricture applies particularly to salves and ointments containing sulphonamides for local control of surface infections (excepting eye infections – see above). Many effective germicides such as ethyl alcohol (q.v.) are available to prevent the infection of a cut or bruise, but few drugs apart from the sulphonamides can control fatal systemic diseases such as meningococcal meningitis (cerebrospinal fever).

Other possible but rare side effects include goitre and hypothyroidism, arthritis and central nervous disturbances.

The sulphonamides are usually administered orally, but they can be injected. Trade names: Sulphadiazine; Sulphamerazine; Trisulphapyrimidine (a mixture: sulphadiazine, sulphamerazine, sulphamethazine); Gantrisin (sulphisoxazole); Gantanol (sulphamethoxazole); Kynex, Midicel (sulphamethoxypyridazine); Madribon (sulphadimethoxine); Sulphasuxidine (succinylsulphathiazole); Sulphathalidine (phthalylsulphathiazole); Thio-sulfil (sulphamethizole); Sulamyd (sulphacetamide).

Testosterone

(Synthesized: Ruzicka and Wettstein, 1935; Butenandt and Hanisch, 1935, Ger.) Trade names: Testoral; (in combination with other compounds) – Andronate, Andrusol-P, Masenate, Neo-hombreol, Sustanon 100, Primoteston Depot, Delatestryl, Tes PP, Oreton propionate (U.S.). Administration: oral, injection.

Classification
The most active male hormone, originally isolated from testicular tissue in crystalline form by Laquen *et al.* (1935), although this was preceded in 1931 by the isolation from 15,000 litres of male urine of the breakdown product androsterone (Butenandt), and subsequently in 1934 of another androgen, dehydro-epiandrosterone (Butenandt and Dannebaum) which was later shown to be produced not from the testis, but from the adrenal (see 'Hormone'). Testosterone is really active only in the ester (see 'Biochemistry') form given usually by injection, although large doses given orally will certainly cause virilization in women. Thus the search for orally active related compounds has been intense, but has been largely unsuccessful.

Other related compounds have been synthesized which show oral activity (methyl testosterone, fluoxymesterone, dehydroiso-androsterone, drostanolone), but these have mainly found application in the palliative treatment of widespread breast cancer ('Therapeutic uses', below). For the androgen derivatives used as anabolic (see 'Metabolism') agents the reader is referred to 'Oxymetholone'.

Therapeutic uses
The main application of the true androgens (as opposed to the anabolic steroids) is in the treatment of androgen deficiency in the body, whether due to failure of the testes or of the pituitary.

Testicular failure is not recognizable until puberty, when the normal changes which should occur (penile growth, increase in height and appearance of body hair) are not seen. Deepening voice, change in distribution of fat and acne which accompany adolescence also fail to occur, and if the condition is not recognized, the further changes which give rise to the typical appearance of the eunuch may take place. If testicular failure arises after puberty, for example by castration, most of the secondary sex characteristics remain, except that libido largely disappears, and impotence often results. It should be made clear, however, that the most common cause of such changes, seen in a greater percentage of the normal male population than is generally realized, is not deficient androgen secretion by the testis, but either stress of the 'rat-race' or frigidity of the sexual partner. Such unfortunate men can frequently exhibit full potency with another partner prepared to give them the mental and physical encouragement and reassurance that they require. Only if they also exhibit impotence in such a situation can the diagnosis of true hormonal failure even be considered, and appropriate treatment instituted.

Another form of hormonal failure amenable to therapy is hypopituitarism with childhood dwarfism, where there is a deficiency not only of androgens but of various other hormones (q.v.) Whatever the cause of the disease, consideration of treatment brings one into an area of considerable debate. Partly at least this is due to the difficulty of ascertaining exactly when puberty occurs; the age of sexual maturation varies considerably, and the clear possibility exists of treating an apparently underdeveloped boy who is merely experiencing a late onset of puberty. The other difference in opinion which significantly influences the practising physician concerns the effect of administered androgens on bone development. Thus it is known that large doses may cause premature cessation of growth at the ends of the long bones. However, this appears to be a matter of dosage, and certainly the use of small quantities of androgen on a continuous basis to cause height increase is well established in complete testicular failure, and in hypopituitarism.

Use of androgens in ageing men to maintain their activities beyond the andropause (the male equivalent of the menopause, which does not occur as suddenly, however) has also been advocated, and here again there is considerable debate, as indeed there appears to be on any subject where sex is involved (see, for example, menopausal therapy under 'Oestradiol', and oral contraceptives under 'Progesterone'). In part no doubt this is an expression of our Puritan ancestry. Nevertheless, it is not yet certain whether treatment with an androgen can be beneficial in maintenance of sexual activity, or for that matter how one could assess the benefit, except in terms of sexual activity. However, there must be many other parameters which are affected by the andropause, for example physical and mental activity, perhaps memory and what could be called, for want of a better word, wisdom. Clearly this is a fruitful field of research for the combined efforts of the endocrinologist and the psychologist, and it may be that in the future we will see preservation of the dignity of old age, rather than the degeneration so graphically pictured by Shakespeare:

> Last scene of all,
> That ends this strange eventful history,
> Is second childishness and mere oblivion,
> Sans teeth, sans eyes, sans taste, sans everything.
> *As You Like It*, Act II, Scene 7

Androgens are also used in the treatment of osteoporosis, where there is a loss of calcium from the bones with consequent weakening of the skeleton, and in the treatment of certain forms of anaemia refractory to the more usual forms of therapy. However, there is reason to believe that this use is more related to their anabolic action and is discussed under 'Oxymetholone'.

Surprisingly, these compounds are used in females also, despite possible virilization, characterized (predictably) by deepening of the voice, growth of facial hair and occasionally development of certain sexual characteristics reminiscent of the male. They are used in menopausal conditions, they are added to oestrogen to diminish the amount of vaginal bleeding when oestrogens are withdrawn, and to cause an increased feeling of well-being and vigour at this otherwise distressing time. Androgens also cause decrease in the size of secondary deposits in about twenty-five per cent of cases of widespread breast cancer. Their mechanism of action in this condition is largely unknown, although it is presumably to antagonize the action of the oestrogen which is required for breast tumour growth in about sixty per cent of cases. However, recently, one compound, drostanolone propionate, which is associated with a higher degree of regression (decrease in size of deposits) than the other androgens, with a lower incidence of virilization, has been shown specifically to inhibit the uptake of radioactive oestrogen by breast tumour tissues, and to alter the metabolic pathways of the tumour cells in a manner which decreases the available energy for cell growth and division. Yet, even this compound causes regression in only about thirty-five to forty per cent of patients. It is to be hoped that further research in cell chemistry may lead to a better understanding of how the tumour cells work, and consequently to better and more effective treatment.

Side effects

Virilization, due to the use of these compounds in women, is described above. It may be accompanied by baldness of the male type, which is thought to be a specific effect of androgens. Other side effects which occur include oedema, due to salt and water retention which responds to diuretics (q.v.). With some testosterone-related compounds jaundice may occur due to blockage of bile in the fine vessels in the liver, although without obstruction in the larger ducts. The jaundice does not appear to be associated with irreversible or severe damage to the liver cells, and is dose-dependent. In addition it appears to be at least partly due to a cumulative effect of drug therapy. For this reason, courses of treatment are frequently interrupted to allow the body to clear the drug.

Chemistry and physiology

The androgens used in treatment of deficiency due either to hypogonadism, or to hypopituitarism are nearly all testosterone esters, in which the side chain is added to prolong the activity of the administered compound. For oral use, however, methyltestosterone or fluoxymesterone may be used (although the attainment of sexual development with the latter is said to be less complete), and both of these compounds contain the 17 alpha-methyl group which protects them from early inactivation in the liver.

The production of testosterone by the testis, and its control by the pituitary are described under 'Hormone'. It acts on the semeniferous tubules to cause sperm production, and is responsible for the secondary male characteristics. In addition it has an anabolic action, and promotes muscle growth, vigour and well-being; it encourages growth in height. Androgens appear to be specifically active in causing increased production of sebum by sebaceous glands, and this explains the acne which occurs commonly around the time of puberty in the male. The development of anti-androgens (see 'Progesterone') has offered hope to sufferers from this condition, but so far, although these compounds can be shown to be active in, for example, diminishing sexual desire, they have not proved efficacious in treating acne either by oral or topical administration.

The cellular mechanism of action of testosterone is not certain. It must apparently be converted to a closely related compound, 5-alpha-dihydrotestosterone, for activity. It is bound to nuclei in cells of sensitive organs where it increases biosynthesis of nucleic acids (ribonucleic acid, RNA, and deoxyribonucleic acid, DNA), thus indirectly increasing biosynthesis of protein.

Tetracycline

(Stephens, *et al.*, 1952, U.S.) Trade names: Achromycin, Ambramycin, Economycin, Macrocyclin, Steclin, Tetracyn, Tetrex, Totomycin; Ger. – Hostacycline; U.S. – Banmycin, Polycycline; in combination with other drugs – Achromycin V, Mysteclin, Sigmanycin. Administration: oral, and may be injected; also, eye-drops.

Classification

One of a group of chemically-similar antibiotics (q.v.), the first of which, chlortetracycline (trade name: Aureomycin), emerged from an intensive research programme in 1948. Chlortetracycline and oxytetracycline (trade name: Tetramycin) were elaborated by *Streptomyces aureofaciens* and *Streptomyces rimosus*, respectively. Demethylchlortetracycline (trade name: Declomycin), the fourth drug in the group, was derived from a mutant of the former organism. Tetracycline itself was first produced semi-synthetically in that chlortetracycline was modified artificially, but tetracycline was later obtained from yet another strain of *Streptomyces* – a case of the laboratory anticipating nature. Newer synthetic members of the family include methacycline and lymecycline.

The tetracyclines are called broad-spectrum antibiotics because they either kill or inhibit the growth of a wide range of non-resistant ('Chemistry and physiology', below) bacteria, both Gram-negative and Gram-positive (see 'Antibiotic'), as well as other infectious organisms known as rickettsiae and mycoplasmae, and some viruses. All tetracyclines have approximately the same therapeutic uses and side effects.

Therapeutic uses

These antibiotics are the only drugs which can be used against rickettsial infections, a group of rare but usually fatal diseases including Rocky Mountain spotted fever, certain forms of typhus, a form of pox and Q-fever.

Lymphogranuloma venereum, a venereal disease of growing statistical importance, responds well to these agents, as does psittacosis or 'parrot fever'. Certain eye diseases including a serious conjunctivitis and trachoma (often treated with sulphona-mides, q.v.) can usually be cured with a tetracycline. A form of pneumonia caused by a mycoplasma, and bacterial infections of bacillae, including brucellosis, tularaemia (streptomycin, q.v., is preferred) and typhoid fever (chloramphenicol, see 'Anti-biotic', is preferred) can be effectively treated with these drugs. Coccal bacteria (e.g. streptococcus, gonococcus) have tended to become resistant to them, but pneumonia, meningitis, gonor-rhoea and other diseases caused by these organisms may nevertheless respond to therapy with tetracycline. Certain difficult urinary tract infections and some phases of syphilis can also be helped. Under some circumstances, the tetracyclines may be employed against yaws, relapsing fever, gas gangrene (peni-cillin, q.v., is preferred), tuberculosis (with other drugs) and some forms of peritonitis. These compounds are among the few that have proved useful against intestinal amoebiasis.

Patients with chronic lung diseases may benefit if one of these drugs is employed to prevent new infections from complicating the existing conditions. The danger of superinfections ('Side effects', below) limits their use for prophylaxis, however.

Side effects

The tetracyclines have proved to be remarkably safe drugs, but they may nevertheless very occasionally produce untoward reactions which can be extremely dangerous. Like other anti-biotics (see 'Penicillin', 'Streptomycin'), they may produce allergy-like hypersensitivity reactions including skin rashes and sores, fever, blood disorders, localized oedema (excess fluid in body tissues) and anaphylaxis, a condition like shock which can be fatal. Sensitivity to one of these drugs means that the patient is in all probability sensitive to them all.

Gastrointestinal irritation caused by the agents can produce stomach upset, nausea, vomiting and diarrhoea. Intravenous injections with the drugs may be followed by a blockage and swelling in the vein used. Toxic effects occasionally appear as blood disturbances and as a so-called 'sunburn' reaction in which light irritates the skin. Liver and kidney damage has also resulted from the tetracyclines. They may cause discoloration of teeth, particularly in children, because the compounds appear to be deposited in growing teeth, and in bones. None of these agents are safely given to pregnant women, particularly during the early weeks, because they can cross the placenta, and can be deposited in the teeth of the developing foetus.

Superinfections occur when the drugs upset the balance of the micro-organisms which normally inhabit the intestines. Sensitive bacteria are destroyed, opening the way to rapid proliferation of insensitive families. Gastrointestinal superinfections can lead to severe and possibly fatal colitis.

Efforts to reduce possible side effects by use of combinations of drugs with tetracyclines have been generally unsuccessful (see 'Therapeutic uses' for exceptions). Indeed, penicillin appears to be antagonized by these agents in pneumococcal meningitis so that neither compound is effective.

Chemistry and physiology

The drug takes its name from the fact that the molecule contains four hexagonal carbon rings (see 'Biochemistry') with various atoms attached to them. Its chemical behaviour in the body is unknown, and may take different courses in different tissues. There are three hypotheses as to its mechanism of action within cells: (1) The drug molecule firmly binds ions (q.v.) essential to cellular structural development, particularly calcium. This action would contribute to an explanation of the appearance of the drug in teeth and bones. (2) The drug becomes attached to enzymes (q.v.) in the place of the natural molecules, and thus inhibits the catalytic action of the enzymes. (3) The drug interferes with the process of cellular protein synthesis in some undefined manner. Since certain ions and several enzymes are essential to protein synthesis, all three actions could be closely interrelated, but which one occurs first remains uncertain.

Bacteria develop resistance to the tetracyclines as to other antibiotics. Resistant strains may develop some mechanism which enables them to withstand the drugs, but their ability to do so must be inherited, or the result of a mutation.

Thiacetazone. U.S.: Amithiozone

(Jouin and Buu-Hoi, 1946, Fr.) Trade names: Thiazina, Thioparamizone; U.S.: Tibione, Panrone; Ger.: Conteben. Administration: oral.

Classification

The discoverer of the forerunner compound from which thiacetazone evolved was Domagk, a German who had earlier been responsible for the first sulphonamide (q.v.), prontosil. Thiacetazone is distantly related chemically to the sulphonamides. Recent research in this general class of compounds has produced evidence that a compound first synthesized in 1906, known as DPT, also has value in the treatment of leprosy, but produces bacterial resistance quickly. Thiambutosine is another such agent.

Therapeutic uses

Thiacetazone, often in combination with isoniazid (q.v.), is used in the treatment of tuberculosis. It is generally less effective than streptomycin (q.v.), but it may be employed when the patient is sensitive to the antibiotic, or when the causative bacteria have become resistant to it.

The drug is more often used against leprosy, however. Since the discovery during the 1930s that this ancient disease responded to treatment with sulphonamides, it has been controlled and even cured with pharmacotherapy. The most frequently used agent is dapsone, but again, some patients are sensitive to this compound, and resistance to it develops among the causative organisms. Indeed, thiacetazone has occasionally proved more effective than dapsone. Thiambutosine and an even newer drug, lampren, may also be employed clinically.

Tuberculosis and leprosy are caused by species of the family of *Mycobacteria*. Thiacetazone halts the growth of the organisms but, in therapeutically safe doses, does not kill them. After drug treatment, it remains for the body's natural immunological defences to extirpate the bacteria finally.

Side effects

Minor untoward reactions include loss of appetite, vomiting, gastric discomfort, vertigo, headache, eye disturbances and skin eruptions. The latter may be controlled by anti-histamines (see 'Tripelennamine'). Blood disorders, including serious anaemia, fever, excess fluid in the brain, swelling and eruption of membranes in the nose and anus, and liver disorders which often reveal themselves as jaundice are among the more serious side effects. Liver disturbances disappear when the drug is discontinued.

Chemistry and physiology

Thiacetazone is one of a group of sulphur-containing compounds called thiosemicarbazones. It causes abnormal changes in the microscopic appearance of *Mycobacteria*, but its mechanism of action is unknown.

Bacterial resistance to the drug does not appear in test-tube experiments, but for reasons which may have to do with conditions within the host, resistance does develop during clinical use. The manner in which some bacteria withstand the drug while others do not is no more clear than the basic behaviour of the drug.

Tranquillizer

These drugs are relaxants that sedate during the daytime and produce sleep at night. Under this heading, we will consider the minor tranquillizers. The major tranquillizers are represented by chlorpromazine (q.v.) and two other types of agent, haloperidol and reserpine, although the latter is less widely used. The major tranquillizers are employed to control severe psychotic illnesses such as schizophrenia whereas the minor tranquillizers control the symptoms of anxiety.

The barbiturates (see 'Phenobarbitone') were the earliest tranquillizers. In 1954, meprobamate (Equanil, Miltown) was developed. It remains the most popular drug of its chemical class as well as one of the most popular tranquillizers. A new chemical type, the benzodiazepines, was introduced in 1960. Chlordiazepoxide (Librium) was the first, and it has been followed by diazepam (Valium), oxazepam (Serenid, Serax), nitrazepam (Mogadon) and several others.

Meprobamate may be used to control alcoholism, tension headaches, premenstrual tension, motion sickness and insomnia. It can be helpful for relaxation in the first stages of labour. The benzodiazepines are also useful for alcoholism, and they may be used with drugs such as imipramine (q.v.) and phenelzine (q.v.) in the control of more severe mental illnesses. Diazepam has helped some types of epilepsy, and may be used for premedication before surgery, for relief of cerebral palsy and in treatment of tetanus. For tetanus, the agent is always injected, but under most other circumstances, the tranquillizers are taken orally.

These drugs are most popular of course for the treatment of mild anxiety symptoms and related neuroses. Indeed, there is evidence that they have been prescribed as a placebo, a substance supposedly without effect, like sugar, that is intended to make the patient believe he has been treated, in the mistaken belief that the minor tranquillizers are harmless. Chlordiazepoxide and diazepam are prescribed by British doctors more frequently than any other drug.

Like depression (see 'Imipramine'), anxiety is a loose assembly of poorly defined symptoms. The indications of anxiety may include insomnia, vague unfocused fear, real or imaginary loss of security, changes in facial expression, nervous mannerisms, peptic ulcer, ulcerative colitis and asthma. The more severe phobic anxieties that are focused on some place or thing do not respond to the minor tranquillizers.

When the disease state is so vague and dissociated from any clearcut biophysical malfunction, it is doubly hard to determine what errors of metabolism (q.v.) drugs may be correcting. It is known that meprobamate does not affect the peripheral nervous system (see 'Adrenaline'), but that it works in the brain. It depresses the conduction of nervous impulses through nerve cells in the hypothalamus, a brain centre ultimately responsible for the secretion of hormones (q.v.) by endocrine glands such as the pituitary, and a brain tract called the reticular activating net which is responsible for alertness and wakefulness or sleep. Chlordiazepoxide suppresses electrical discharges in the brain region called the limbic system which lies between the hypothalamus and the reticular net, and incorporates part of the latter. The limbic system plays an important but poorly understood role in the regulation of emotion. Thus, the tranquillizers like other psychoactive drugs appear to exert their effects in brain centres associated with both emotion and alertness. Their biochemical actions are not known, however.

Under normal circumstances, meprobamate is a very safe

drug, and the benzodiazepines are only slightly more toxic. None of the minor tranquillizers have been used successfully to commit suicide, which makes them much safer as sleeping pills than the barbiturates. However, acute meprobamate poisoning is known. It appears as low blood pressure, convulsions, coma and death. The only symptoms of acute benzodiazepine poisoning are drowsiness and depression of respiration, blood pressure and pulse rate, though very large doses might also be fatal.

All of the minor tranquillizers are, nevertheless, addictive. Chlordiazepoxide does not produce euphoria, but the evidence on the other compounds is less certain. They can all lead to compulsive use and physical dependence. Withdrawal from meprobamate can cause psychotic behaviour, convulsions and coma, and has even been fatal. With chlordiazepoxide, withdrawal symptoms include seizures, convulsions, depression, agitation, insomnia and loss of appetite. These symptoms may appear a week or two after the drugs have been discontinued. They are infrequent, however, and seldom occur with moderate doses.

A few patients have displayed allergy-like reactions to the minor tranquillizers. Meprobamate has caused blood disorders and even rare cases of aplastic anaemia. If taken with alcohol (see 'Ethyl alcohol'), the drugs can disturb perception and motor function. Benzodiazepines greatly enhance the actions of barbiturates, phenothiazines (see 'Chlorpromazine'), MAO inhibitors (see 'Phenelzine') and tricyclic anti-depressants (see 'Imipramine'). They should not be given to patients with glaucoma because they tend to increase the interocular fluid pressure that underlies the disease. In old people, the tranquillizers much enhance drowsiness and lethargy, but such is their general effect that no one taking any of these agents should drive.

Tripelennamine

(Yonkman, *et al.*, 1946, U.S.) Trade name: Pyribenzamine. Administration: oral, but can be injected.

Classification
One of the earliest of a large group of synthetic agents called collectively anti-histamines. All such drugs have a chemical

similarity ('Chemistry and physiology', below), but they fall into several structural subcategories. Although these compounds each antagonize some of the actions of histamine, a natural local hormone (q.v., and below), their range of effects varies. In addition to tripelennamine, the more familiar anti-histamines include diphenhydramine (trade name: Benadryl), dimenhydrinate (trade name: Dramamine), thonzylamine (trade name: Anahist), chlorpheniramine (trade name: Chlortrimeton) and cyclazine (trade name: Marzine).

Therapeutic uses

Tripelennamine and the other anti-histamines are perhaps most widely employed for the control of symptoms arising from common allergies such as hay fever. An allergy is a reaction to dust, pollen or some other foreign substance (antigen) which causes mobilization of some or all of the immunological defence mechanisms. The symptoms include sneezing, coughing, itching and, in more extreme cases, difficulty in breathing and a sharp decrease in blood pressure characteristic of shock. Only the more superficial reactions can be controlled by anti-histamines. Asthma, for example, which is thought to be in some cases an allergic reaction, is not greatly helped by these agents, though a pre-asthmatic cough in children may be ameliorated. Allergic skin conditions often respond to the drugs, but if they are applied at the point where irritation has occurred (that is, to the skin locally), the agents themselves can cause an allergic reaction. Localized excess fluids in body tissues (angioneurotic oedema) are in some cases evidence of allergic reaction and can be reduced by the use of anti-histamines. The drugs also aid the itching caused by insect bites and poison ivy.

Tripelennamine is less effective than other anti-histamines such as diphenhydramine and dimenhydrinate in the control or prevention of motion sickness. Drugs useful for this purpose may also be employed to prevent post-operative vomiting and nausea and the vomiting of pregnancy.

All of the anti-histamines may be used to control symptoms of parkinsonism (see 'L-Dopa') and as hypnotics (see 'Phenobarbitone'). They also have a local anaesthetic action which contributes to their power to stop itching, but again there is danger that the agent itself will produce an allergic reaction.

There is no evidence that these drugs help to *cure* a common cold. However, they may produce some reduction in symptoms and thus afford subjective relief.

Side effects

Individual responses to compounds of this type vary widely, but all of the drugs can produce some undesirable effects. Usually they are not serious and will disappear when the drug is stopped. Excessive dosage can cause severe, sometimes fatal poisoning, however, especially in children. Symptoms include hallucinations, loss of muscular control, convulsions, coma and cardiorespiratory collapse. Treatment for anti-histamine poisoning depends on the symptoms, but it is more frequently physical (for example, artificial respiration) rather than pharmacological.

The most common side effect produced by this class of agent is sedation. Indeed, the sedative effect may be useful for the control of itching or in the prevention of motion sickness. Tripelennamine is less sedative than other anti-histamines, but it is nevertheless unwise to drive after using any of these compounds.

Other mild reactions can include loss of appetite, vomiting, gastrointestinal discomfort, constipation *or* diarrhoea, dryness of the mouth, urinary frequency or the reverse, palpitation, a fall in blood pressure, heaviness and weakness in the hands.

Allergy-like reactions have been referred to under 'Therapeutic uses'. More severe hypersensitivity effects appear rarely as blood disorders.

Chemistry and physiology

All anti-histamines share with the natural substance, histamine, the chemical nucleus: $-CH_2CH_2N=$. It seems probable, therefore, that this nucleus is the site in the molecule which causes the action to occur, and that it does so by binding to an effector molecule on or within cells. Thus the drugs compete with histamine at such effector molecules, and antagonize the natural substance. However, because both histamine and the anti-histamines display different and in some cases contradictory actions in different tissues, it is thought that the effector molecules may also differ. In any case, they have not been identified so that the basic mechanism of action of both the local hormone and the synthetic antagonists is unclear.

Histamine is synthesized by mast cells, a distinctive type of cell found primarily in connective tissue. They also synthesize the natural anti-coagulant, heparin (q.v.). Histamine is released upon local irritation by an antigen, or by a cut, bruise or bite. Among other effects, histamine tends to lower blood pressure in man by allowing the cells which form capillaries and other small blood vessels to separate slightly, thus opening the vessels more widely. In the process, the blood plasma (blood minus red cells) and certain substances dissolved in it more readily escape so that fluid collects in the tissue, causing swelling and pain. Another action of histamine occurs at the ends of nerves so that itching occurs. In yet another action, the substance causes an increase in the secretion of pepsin and hydrochloric acid by cells in the stomach; this effect is the only one which appears not to be affected by anti-histamines, suggesting that the receptor molecules in the secretory cells of the stomach differ in such a way that they cannot bind the drug despite its chemical resemblance to histamine.

In the bronchioles, the tiny air passages in the lungs, histamine appears to mediate constriction. Thus it is implicated in an asthmatic attack.

As a result of the appearance of histamine, other substances are also released into the affected tissues. There is evidence that histamine is only one, though perhaps the first, in a cascade effect which produces the symptoms of inflammation common in allergies, minor wounds and some diseases (see 'Aspirin'). The anti-histamines may have some limited effect against an asthmatic attack, probably because histamine does play a role in producing it, but the inefficacy of these drugs is thought to be due to the presence in the lungs of other natural substances released by cells under the influence of histamine.

Although it is their specifically histamine-antagonizing effects which give the drugs their usefulness in combating the symptoms of allergies, their sedative effect and their value against motion sickness seem to arise from actions having nothing to do with histamine. In this respect, the name anti-histamine appears to be irrelevant if not misapplied. Wakefulness, balance (disturbances of which underlie motion sickness) and the nervous control which is impaired by Parkinson's disease are all functions of brain centres. The drugs evidently act at these centres, but the manner is unknown.

Vitamin

Literally: amine (or nitrogen-containing compound) of life. The name arose from the realization that thiamine (vitamin B_1), the first vitamin to be identified chemically, contained nitrogen. A modern textbook gives the definition: 'a substance that is essential for the maintenance of normal metabolic (see "Metabolism") functions but which is not synthesized in the body and therefore must be furnished from an exogenous source.'* At least two hundred years ago, doctors became aware that certain

* Goodman and Gilman, *op. cit.*, p. 1649.

possibly fatal diseases occurred because some element was missing from an otherwise adequate diet. Perhaps the first conscious attempt to prevent disease by supplying such a substance was that instituted by the British Navy in 1804 when a daily ration of lemon or lime juice to prevent scurvy became compulsory.

In the table overleaf, all known vitamins are listed along with their common sources, the deficiency diseases to which their lack gives rise, the causes of the deficiency, the coenzyme or prosthetic group (see 'Enzyme') in which they function and their normal metabolic and physiological functions. Note that the list is organized in accordance with the letter and number sequence of the 'popular' names, and that descriptive chemical names do not appear. Excepting in the cases of Niacin and Decavitamin preparations, trade names of vitamins are the same as their common chemical names. In this respect, they differ from other drugs (see 'Introduction') which have common and descriptive chemical names as well as trade names. The list also contains four substances – choline, inositol, para-amino-benzoic acid (PABA) and vitamin P – which are included because textbooks describe them with vitamins as a matter of custom, although they are improperly so classified for reasons given in the table.

Popular name	Common chemical name	Common source*	Deficiency diseases	Reasons for deficiency	Coenzyme or prosthetic group	Metabolic and physiological functions*
Vitamin A₁†‡ A₂†‡	Retinol 3-Dehydro-retinol	Carrots Green vegetables	Night blindness Softening and destruction of cornea and conjunctiva of eye Dermatitis Kidney stones Diarrhoea Defects in nerves, bones Widespread infection	Diet Malabsorption: (1) disorders of fat absorption (2) liver disorders	Retinene	Formation of visual pigments§ Stimulation of epithelial mucopolysaccharide synthesis Synthesis of gluco-corticoids (see 'Hormone') Normal growth
B-vitamins§ Vitamin B₁‡	Thiamine	Yeast Liver Rice polishings	Beriberi Alcoholic neuritis Neuritis of pregnancy Cardiovascular disease of nutritional origin	Diet Malabsorption due to gastrointestinal disorders	Thiamine pyrophosphate	Intermediary metabolism of carbohydrates
Vitamin B₂‡	Riboflavin	Milk Yeast Liver	Corneal destruction General inflammation of mucous membranes (Usually associated with pellagra)	Diet	Riboflavin phosphate (FMN) Flavin adenine dinucleotide (FAD)‡	Oxidation-reduction of intracellular respiratory proteins in electron transport system§

Niacin (B3)	Nicotinic acid	Liver Yeast	Pellagra	Diet	Nicotinamide adenine dinucleotide (NAD) Nicotinamide adenine dinucleotide phosphate (NADP)	As above, prior to FAD in systems§
Vitamin B6‡	Pyridoxine Pyridoxal Pyridox-amine	Liver Yeast	Skin lesions Convulsions Hypochromic anaemia (see Note on B12) Peripheral neuritis from isoniazid (q.v.) treatment	Diet	Pyridoxal phosphate Pyridoxamine phosphate	Conversions of certain amino acids to others
Vitamin B12§‡	Cyanoco-balamin	Liver Heart Kidney Bivalves: clams, oysters	Pernicious anaemia Demyelinization	Malabsorption: (1) absence of gastric intrinsic factor (2) intestinal damage	Deoxyadenosyl B12	Normal synthesis of formed-elements of blood Normal production of all epithelial cells Formation and maintenance of substance which may serve to insulate nerves from each other (myelin) Normal synthesis of nucleo-proteins Normal growth

Popular name	Common chemical name	Common source*	Deficiency diseases	Reasons for deficiency	Coenzyme or prosthetic group	Metabolic and physiological functions*
Folic acid§‡	Pteroyl-monogluta-mic acid	Yeast Liver Green vegetables	Megaloblastic anaemia	Diet Malabsorption due to intestinal damage Malutilization: (1) caused by drugs (2) absence of B_{12}	Tetrahydrofolic acid (various) forms	Normal synthesis of DNA·RNA precursors (purines and pyrimidines) Conversions of certain amino acids to others Use of various essential metabolites
None	Pantothenic acid	Ubiquitous	Only experimental	Only induced experimentally	Coenzyme A	Transfer of 2-carbon fragments in carbohydrate metabolism, especially in form: acetyl-Coenzyme A
None	Biotin	Food Intestinal bacteria	Only experimental	As above	Biotin	Fixation of CO_2
None	Choline	Biosynthesized by human cells			None	Lipotropic agent; i.e. contributes to liver metabolism of fat Precursor of acetylcholine, nerve-impulse transmitter (see 'Atropine')
None	Inositol	Biosynthesized by human cells			None	Unknown

Vitamin	Chemical name	Sources	Deficiency disease	Cause of deficiency	(Toxicity)	Metabolic function
None	Para-amino-benzoic acid (PABA)	Cannot be utilized directly by mammals. Must be ingested as part of folic acid molecule. No evidence that it is required by human beings.				
Vitamin C‡	Ascorbic acid	Citrus fruit Green vegetables	Scurvy Failure to form and maintain collagen§ Haemorrhage from capillary leaks Bone lesions Degeneration of teeth and gums	Diet	None known	Oxidation-reduction and cellular respiration§ Metabolism of excess tyrosine to tryptophan (both essential amino acids) Carbohydrate metabolism Possible biosynthesis of adrenocorticoids (see 'Hormone') Biosynthesis of galactosamine from glucosamine (sugar-aminos essential to formation and maintenance of connective tissue)
Vitamin D₂†‡§ D₃†‡§	Calciferol Activated 7-dehydro cholesterol	Sunshine Fish liver oils (esp. cod)	Rickets (in children) Osteomalacia (in adults) Infantile tetany	Diet Inadequate sunlight Malabsorption: (1) hepatic disease (2) disfunction of bile mechanisms	None known	Ca and P absorption from intestinal tract; deposition and resorption of bone; kidney function in (relation to parathyroid hormone) May act like a hormone (q.v.) to permit expression of specific genes

Popular name	Common chemical name	Common source*	Deficiency diseases	Reasons for deficiency	Coenzyme or prosthetic group	Metabolic and physiological functions*
Vitamin E	α, β, γ, δ, ε, ζ-tocopherol	Wheat germ oil	In sub-primate mammals: Sterility Foetal death Muscular dystrophy Disturbances of fat metabolism In man and primates: 'Vitamin E' anaemia	Probably diet	Unknown, though chemically similar to Enzyme Q	Probably participates in regulation of biosynthesis of the haem group, the iron-containing molecule which binds (or releases) oxygen and gives the red colouring to the larger haemoglobin molecule of which it is a part
Vitamin K₁ K₂ K₃†	Phytonadione Menadione	Many foods Intestinal bacteria	Increased bleeding tendencies	Diet Drugs that inhibit intestinal bacteria Malabsorption All rare	Unknown, but possibly a prosthetic group	Essential to biosynthesis of blood-clotting factors: prothrombin, factors VII, IX and X (see 'Dicoumarol' and 'Heparin') Oxidation-reduction and cellular respiration§
Vitamin P	Flavonoids	Citrus fruit Paprika	Unknown	Non-existent	Unknown	Unknown

*Listing is incomplete. †Toxic reactions possible from high doses or in certain abnormal states,
‡Included in decavitamin preparations. §See Notes to the Table, pp. 247-9 ff.
N.B.: All B-vitamins and Vitamins C and P are soluble in water, Vitamins A, D, E and K are soluble in fat.

Notes to the table

Vitamin A

The visual cycle, in which retinol participates after it has been converted in the body to retinene, is an extremely complex sequence of chemical events, the purpose of which is to convert light energy into a nervous impulse to flow from the retina along the optic nerve to the appropriate centre at the back of the brain. There are two principal chemicals in the retina both of which are required for the visual cycle to occur, and in both of which retinene is a prosthetic group:

$$\text{Retinene} + \text{opsin} = \text{rhodopsin}$$
$$\text{Retinene} + \text{photopsin} = \text{iodopsin}$$

Each of these end products is associated with one of the two types of light-sensitive retinal cells. Rhodopsin exists in the rods, which are sensitive to dimmer light towards the violet end of the spectrum, whereas iodopsin occurs in the cones, which are sensitive to brighter light towards the red end. Thus, rhodopsin and iodopsin are called visual pigments.

How this vitamin performs its other metabolic and physiological functions is still unclear. Various hypotheses have emerged to explain effects of the vitamin on mucous formation, on membranes surrounding cells and cellular organelles and on RNA synthesis, but none have yet proven to be entirely satisfactory.

B-vitamins

These substances are grouped together because they are water-soluble, and were originally thought to have been available naturally in yeast and liver.

Vitamin B_2

'Oxidation-reduction of intracellular respiratory proteins in electron transport system.' This note should be read in conjunction with the entry on 'Biochemistry'. It is noted there that a major part of metabolic (see 'Metabolism') activity is devoted to the formation of energy-storage molecules, ATP. To this end, food is catabolized step by step with the release of CO_2 and H_2O. The process does not end there, however, for the largest increment of stored energy derives from oxidation of the end products of food catabolism. Oxidation is a chemical event in which one of three atomic changes occurs within the molecule undergoing the oxidation: (1) an atom of oxygen is added to it; (2) an atom of hydrogen is removed from it (both (1) and (2) occur more or less simultaneously); (3) electrons are removed from it. Reduction is the reverse chemical event; i.e. an atom of oxygen is removed, a hydrogen atom is added, or electrons are added.

Oxidation can occur anaerobically; i.e. in the absence of oxygen. Oxidations in yeasts, for example, are anaerobic, which explains why alcoholic fermentations in the presence of yeast should take place in air-tight containers. Human cells, especially muscle cells, engage in anaerobic oxidation, but there is a limit, for two reasons: (1) in human cells, one of the end products of anaerobic oxidation is a sugar derivative, lactate, the salt of lactic acid, which cannot be further broken down without oxygen and is toxic in excess. (2) Aerobic oxidation (in the presence of oxygen) supplies significantly more energy in the form of additional molecules of ATP than does anaerobic oxidation. Because anaerobic oxidation is more frequently the mode in unicellular organisms and aerobic oxidation in multicellular organisms, it may in passing be reasonable to suggest that the latter reflects an evolutionary forward step, a hypothesis supported by the fact that life is thought to have begun in the sea.

Aerobic oxidation requires the presence of atmospheric oxygen (O_2), which is one of the principal reasons why we breathe. In cells, the mechanism by means of which end products of food catabolism are combined with O_2 to release energy (as well as CO_2 and H_2O) is called electron transport. As the name implies, the mechanism moves electrons and protons, not molecules. It consists of substances such as FMN, FAD, NAD and NADP which can accept and release electrons and protons; in other words, they can engage in oxidation-reduction cycles (called 'redox'). Molecules of these respiratory proteins appear to be literally lined up next to each other in the correct order within the membranous walls of intracellular organelles called mitochondria. There they are juxtaposed appropriately to H, ADP, ATP and O_2 in the intra-mitochondrial fluids. NAD, NADP and the flavins appear early in the electron-transport mechanism and transfer hydrogen atoms which are then ionized (see 'Ion') to hydrogen ions (H^+) and electrons. These pass down a chain of three or possibly more cytochromes (molecules which have a colour), the last one of which passes two electrons to O_2. This oxygen then picks up two spare hydrogen ions with the formation of water. Energy from the redox transactions is used to form ATP molecules from ADP molecules. Because formation of ATP from ADP occurs by the addition of phosphate to the latter, the whole aerobic respiratory process is known as oxidative phosphorylation (see 'Aspirin').

Niacin (see note on vitamin B_2, above)

Vitamin B_{12} and Folic acid
The metabolic functions of these two vitamins are intimately inter-related. Broadly speaking, folic acid may be said to be more fundamental because the coenzyme, tetrahydrofolic acid, of which it is an essential part, participates in metabolic functions which must occur prior to the point at which vitamin B_{12} enters the process. Yet in the absence of the latter, folic acid may be inadequately utilized so that a deficiency of this vitamin also appears to exist.

Pernicious anaemia, for the prevention and cure of which vitamin B_{12} is essential, is a type of megaloblastic anaemia. Megaloblasts are deformed cellular precursors of formed elements of the blood, namely, leucocytes (white blood cells), erythrocytes (red blood cells, RBC) and platelets (cells which play a role in blood clotting, see 'Dicoumarol' and 'Heparin', and also in immunological defence). Thus in megaloblastic anaemias, these blood elements are also deformed. Non-megaloblastic anaemias include diseases such as aplastic anaemia and some forms of haemolytic (i.e., the rupturing of haemoglobin-containing RBC) anaemia. Anaemia can also be caused by malformation of RBC due to infection or genetic error, by iron deficiency (hypochromocytic anaemia) and of course by haemorrhage.

One major difference between vitamin B_{12} and folic acid is that the former is essential for the formation and maintenance of the lipo-protein (i.e. protein plus a fat-like moiety combined in one molecule), myelin, which surrounds and protects major nerve cells throughout the body, and plays a role in the normal intraneuronal transmission of nervous impulses. Thus, treatment of megaloblastic anaemia with folic acid alone may, if the patient has pernicious anaemia due to vitamin B_{12} deficiency, lead to cure of the anaemia but with development of demyelinization and irreparable neurological lesions.

Note that malabsorption of vitamin B_{12} from the intestinal tract may be caused by the absence of a substance called gastric intrinsic factor. This is a molecule in the stomach lining, formed by the cells, which has not been identified chemically. Without it, however, the vitamin will not be absorbed through the intestinal wall, unless massive doses are given.

Vitamin C
Collagen, the formation and maintenance of which depends upon an adequate supply of vitamin C, is a protein and one of the major non-cellular constituents of connective tissue.

For an explanation of the oxidation-reduction role of this vitamin, see vitamin B_2, above.

Vitamin D
The two types of this vitamin are popularly labelled D_2 and D_3 respectively because the original vitamin, D_1, was found to be a mixture of calciferol and activated 7-dehydrocholesterol.

Parathyroid hormone is secreted by the parathyroid gland. The hormone (q.v.) is concerned with deposition and, more particularly, reabsorption of calcium and phosphorus in bone. Vitamin D has similar functions, but orientated towards calcium deposition. Thus, in many specific metabolic functions, the two substances have opposite effects so that the net result is attained by means of a balance between them. Vitamin D's action in promoting calcium absorption from the gut is also useful in the treatment of a condition called hypoparathyroidism in which the parathyroid is secreting too little hormone.

Vitamin K
For an explanation of the oxidation-reduction role of this vitamin, see vitamin B_2, above.

The discovery, purification and synthesis of vitamins has contributed one of the brightest chapters in medical history. Deficiency diseases such as scurvy, rickets, beriberi, pellagra and pernicious anaemia can be prevented, or cured when they do appear. Symptoms such as alcoholic neuritis and the neuritis of pregnancy which occur because of dietary deficiencies resulting from special circumstances can also be prevented or cured. Although some deficiency diseases remain, such as kwashiorkor which afflicts millions of children in underdeveloped tropical countries, their causes are usually known, and the cure waits upon a general improvement in the diet of affected populations. In the case of kwashiorkor, the solution is not a vitamin, but more protein. Although the record is by no means perfect, especially among lower income families, on the whole these illnesses have been banished from the developed countries by adequate diet and vitamins.

How ironic, therefore, that among the world's better-fed peoples, vitamins are perhaps second only to aspirin (q.v.) as the universal panacea. They have been taken for everything from hang-nail to bubonic plague; not infrequently, they are prescribed by physicians almost as freely as they are bought over the counter by the public. These doctors at least have an excuse: the vitamins cannot do harm, however large the dose, excepting for vitamins A, D and K_3 (see table), and they might do some good; without vitamins, some doctors argue, they might have to find some other potentially more harmful substance to satisfy the millions of indiscriminate pill takers among us.

But the physicians know, even if the public refuses to accept, that the average inhabitant of Great Britain, the United States and every other developed part of the globe gets perfectly adequate amounts of all vitamins in his usual diet. Only minute quantities are required. There are important exceptions: pregnant and lactating women, chronic alcoholics, sufferers from certain infections and from cancer probably require supplementary doses of vitamins because their conditions make additional demands which often cannot be met from a normal diet. Crash dieters, too, would do well to watch their vitamin intake if they insist on adhering to some purgatorial food regimens sometimes popular with certain discontented, overfed individuals. Vegetarians may need supplements of the more important B-vitamins, particularly B_1, niacin and B_{12}. Infants may require vitamins, especially vitamin K and vitamin B_{12}, for a few days after birth.

As to the use of ascorbic acid to prevent colds, considerable controversy was stirred up in 1970 when Linus Pauling, American biochemist and Nobel Prize winner, argued that very large doses of Vitamin C will prevent the common cold and may reduce its symptoms. Pauling does not attempt to explain how the vitamin achieves such desirable effects, and his evidence that it does is by no means universally accepted. For example, it has been suggested that if doses are taken as pills with unusual amounts of water or other liquids to wash them down, the liquids rather than the vitamin might be controlling cold symptoms. However, vitamin C is water-soluble and probably harmless in that the body excretes what it cannot use. For once, the individual may feel free to experiment.

Most vitamins and multivitamin preparations have no value whatsoever to the average normal individual, though of course they do for anyone who is in any respect undernourished. Vitamin A, vitamin D and vitamin K, it is worth repeating, can be dangerously toxic in large doses. The cure for vitamin poisoning is simplicity itself, however: stop taking vitamins.

Index of Diseases and Disease States

(Including natural conditions such as: Abortion; Childbirth, induction of; Contraception.)